D0875463

CONSUMER VOICE AND CHOICE IN LONG-TERM CARE

About the Editors

Suzanne R. Kunkel, PhD, is the director of Scripps Gerontology Center and professor in the Department of Sociology and Gerontology at Miami University. Dr. Kunkel has 20 years of experience in gerontological research and teaching and has published extensively on long-term care. Her research includes federally funded projects designed to develop and evaluate innovations in homecare. She has been principal investigator or co–principal investigator on three consumer direction projects, including a current study of quality in consumer direction in programs funded by the Robert Wood Johnson Foundation and the Assistant Secretary for Planning and Evaluation at the U.S. Department of Health and Human Services.

Valerie Wellin, BA, is a senior research assistant at Scripps Gerontology Center at Miami University. She previously served as a staff research associate at the Department of Social and Behavioral Sciences, University of California–San Francisco. Before that she worked with a software company that developed products for the health care sector. Wellin has experience as a researcher, co-author, and editor of published articles and reports in the field of long-term care, nursing facilities, and home healthcare. She also has had professional training as a pastry chef.

Consumer Voice and Choice in Long-Term Care

Edited by

Suzanne R. Kunkel and Valerie Wellin

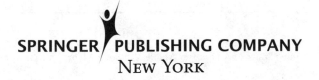

SPRINGER PUBLISHING COMPANY
NEW YORK

Springer Publishing Company, Inc.
11 West 42nd Street
New York, NY 10036

Acquisitions Editor: Sheri W. Sussman
Managing Editor: Mary Ann McLaughlin
Production Editor: Judi Rohrbaugh
Cover Design: Joanne E. Honigman
Typeset by TechBooks

06 07 08 09 10/ 5 4 3 2 1

Library of Congress Cataloging-in-Publication Data

Consumer voice and choice in long-term care / edited by Suzanne R. Kunkel
and Valerie Wellin.
    p. cm.
    Includes some papers presented at a conference organized by the Scripps
Gerontology Center.
    Includes bibliographical references and index.
    ISBN 0-8261-0210-7 (alk. paper)
  1. Older people–Care–United States–Congresses.   2. Caregivers–United
States–Congresses.   3. Consumer behavior–United States–Congresses.
I. Kunkel, Suzanne.   II. Wellin, Valerie.

HQ1064.U5C611375   2006
362.610973—dc22

2006013631

Printed in the United States of America by Maple-Vail Book Manufacturing Group.

Contents

PART II. Consumer Voice

PART III. Policy Issues and Moral and
Legal Challenges

Contributors

Robert A. Applebaum, PhD
Director of the Ohio Long-Term
  Care Research Project, Scripps
  Gerontology Center
Professor, Department of Sociology
  and Gerontology
Miami University
Oxford, Ohio

Barbara Bowers, PhD, RN
Interim Associate Dean for
  Research and Sponsored
  Programs
Helen Denne Schulte Professor
University of Wisconsin-Madison,
  School of Nursing
Madison, Wisconsin

Susan Chapman, PhD
Assistant Adjunct Professor
Department of Social and
  Behavioral Sciences
University of California–San
  Francisco
San Francisco, California

Elias S. Cohen, JD, MPA
Attorney and Consultant
Wynnewood, Pennsylvania

Shawn L. Davis, MGS
Seniors' Resource Center
Denver, Colorado

Farida K. Ejaz, PhD
Senior Research Scientist II
The Margaret Blenkner Research
  Institute
Benjamin Rose
Cleveland, Ohio

Sarah L. Esmond, MS
Project Manager
Center for the Study of Cultural
  Diversity in Healthcare (CDH)
University of Wisconsin Medical
  School
Madison, Wisconsin

Kathleen Fox, MEd
Senior Research Analyst I
The Margaret Blenkner Research
  Institute
Benjamin Rose
Cleveland, Ohio

Lisa Groger, PhD
Research Fellow, Scripps
  Gerontology Center
Professor, Department of
  Sociology and Gerontology
Miami University
Oxford, Ohio

Elizabeth Holloway, PhD
Professor of Psychology
PhD in Leadership and Change
  Program
Antioch University
Yellow Springs, Ohio

Sandra Howell White, PhD
Senior Policy Analyst
Center for State Health Policy
Rutgers University
New Brunswick, New Jersey

**Marshall B. Kapp, JD, MPH,
  FCLM**
Garwin Distinguished Professor of
  Law and Medicine
Southern Illinois University School
  of Law
Carbondale, Illinois

Suzanne R. Kunkel, PhD
Director, Scripps Gerontology
  Center
Professor, Department of
  Sociology and Gerontology
Miami University
Oxford, Ohio

Kevin J. Mahoney, PhD
National Program Director, Cash
  and Counseling Demonstration
  and Evaluation

Associate Professor
Boston College Graduate School of
  Social Work
Chestnut Hill, Massachusetts

Kathryn B. McGrew, PhD
Research Fellow, Scripps
  Gerontology Center
Associate Professor, Department
  of Sociology and Gerontology
Miami University
Oxford, Ohio

Ian Matt Nelson, MGS
Research Associate–Level II,
  Scripps Gerontology Center
Miami University
Oxford, Ohio

Robert Newcomer, PhD
Professor of Medical Sociology,
  Department of Social and
  Behavioral Sciences
Associate Director of the Center for
  Personal Assistance Services
University of California–San
  Francisco
San Francisco, California

Sally Norton, RN, PhD
Assistant Professor
University of Rochester, School of
  Nursing
Rochester, New York

Winifred Quinn, MA
Research Analyst
Center for State Health Policy
Rutgers University
New Brunswick, New Jersey

Susan C. Reinhard, RN, PhD
Professor and Co-Director
Center for State Health Policy
Rutgers University
New Brunswick, New Jersey

Teresa Scherzer, PhD
Assistant Adjunct Professor
Department of Social and
   Behavioral Sciences
University of California–San
   Francisco
San Francisco, California

Dorothy Schur, BA
Research Analyst
The Margaret Blenkner Research
   Institute
Benjamin Rose
Cleveland, Ohio

Mark Sciegaj, PhD, MPH
Associate Professor of Public Policy
   and Management
Director–The RoseMary B. Fuss
   Center for Research on Aging and
   Intergenerational Studies
Lasell College
Newton, Massachusetts

Kristin Simone, MM
Deputy Program Director, Cash
   and Counseling Demonstration
   and Evaluation
Boston College Graduate School of
   Social Work
Chestnut Hill, Massachusetts

Robyn I. Stone, DrPH
Executive Director
Institute for the Future of
   Aging Services
American Association of Homes
   and Services for the Aging
Washington, DC

Jane K. Straker, PhD
Director of Policy, Ohio Long-Term
   Care Research Project, Scripps
   Gerontology Center
Miami University
Oxford, Ohio

Gwen C. Uman, RN, PhD
Partner
Vital Research, LLC
Los Angeles, California

Chris Wellin, PhD
Research Fellow, Scripps
   Gerontology Center
Assistant Professor, Department
   of Sociology and Gerontology
Miami University
Oxford, Ohio

Carol J. Whitlatch, PhD
Assistant Director for Research
The Margaret Blenkner Research
   Institute
Benjamin Rose
Cleveland, Ohio

Acknowledgments

The editors would like to thank the Robert Wood Johnson Foundation for helping to support this effort, particularly in allowing the event that was our inspiration for this volume to happen. We would also like to thank Helvi Gold for her early efforts that got this project off the ground and Sheri W. Sussman for her work in keeping it afloat. Finally, thanks must also go to Robert Applebaum and Chris Wellin for their never-flagging help and moral and technical support during difficult times.

Introduction

Consumer voice and choice have emerged as important and timely factors in (and arguably a wholly different approach to) the design and delivery of long-term care services to elderly and disabled populations. Opportunity for consumers to provide input about their services within the traditional system is a defining element of consumer voice. Hearing from consumers about the quality of, and their satisfaction with, their services has become an essential component of quality management in many sectors of long-term care. Providing service delivery options so that long-term care consumers can truly have choice has required more fundamental changes to the long-term care system. Consumer direction is an innovative service model which emphasizes that autonomy, choice, and less restricted access to services and support are rights of long-term care recipients rather than simply value-added benefits.

Greater involvement and control by consumers in directing and assessing their own care is timely, as this approach, which began with a younger disabled population, has now taken root in the older cohorts including our current seniors and the aging baby-boom generation. Publicly funded consumer-directed programs continue to proliferate. Based on a recent survey of 40 states, three-fourths of those states now offer consumer-directed home- and community-based services for older people; 20 states offer two or more consumer-directed options within their home-care system for older adults (Infeld, 2004). Cash and Counseling, the most fully developed and fully articulated model of consumer direction, is currently being implemented in 15 states. In Cash and Counseling programs, consumers hire and supervise their own workers, direct their own services, and manage their own purchasing plans. Participants receive assistance with these tasks from fiscal intermediary agencies, support brokers/counselors, and, if appropriate, authorized representatives.

What will this emergent approach to long-term care require of its many and varied stakeholders? In short, a great deal. To insure the active role of consumers in the assessing of services and programs, academic and agency-based researchers will need a variety of new and retooled instruments and strategies. Consumer-centered valid and reliable instruments, and effective data collection approaches, are crucial if consumer voice is to be heard in the design and evaluation of quality of care delivered to a vulnerable or at-risk population. Commitment to a new model of service delivery—with all that implies, and by all those involved in the design and implementation of long-term services—is essential. Program administrators, clinical and social service personnel, and other direct-care workers all play crucial roles in making consumer voice and choice a reality. Ensuring their awareness of, commitment to, and role in this innovative approach will be crucial to its success. Policy makers and agency leaders are facing ideological, political, and pragmatic challenges in supporting the shift to consumer-centered service delivery.

This book is intended to serve as a resource as the field of long-term services for older adults increases its commitment to consumer empowerment. This volume describes current research, practice, and critical thought related to consumer voice and choice in long-term care. We envision a broad target audience for this publication, including gerontology, health care and social science students, practitioners/professionals who work in the long-term care industry, policymakers, researchers, and a growing number of people seeking to take an active (even proactive) role in their own care or in the care of others who are close to them.

This book was inspired and informed by a conference—"The Consumer Voice and Choice Conference," which was organized by the Scripps Gerontology Center, and sponsored in part by the Robert Wood Johnson Foundation. In recognizing the evolving and expanding role of consumers in long-term care, the editors of this book have used the conference as a springboard to further explore consumer direction in long-term care. Topics include approaches to capturing and measuring consumer satisfaction and quality, case management, quality improvement, and decision making and planning. Some of the chapters in this book are based on presentations that took place at this conference; other chapters have been added to give a more comprehensive view of the topic.

The book is organized in three parts. Part I, "Consumer Choice," includes factors that may influence an individual's role in planning for their own long-term care needs, the extent to which an older person wishes to be involved in their long-term care, their preferences for service models and for control over specific types of services. This section also describes consumer direction as a model of long-term care service delivery. One chapter describes the Cash and Counseling initiative; another discusses the challenges facing case managers as they shift their role to supporting self-directed consumers. This section also offers a chapter that focuses on the well-being of workers in consumer-driven home care, and assesses a state initiative that helps nursing home residents return to the community by giving consumers and their families information about their long-term care options.

Part II, "Consumer Voice," explores the value of, and approaches to, ascertaining the needs, preferences, and perspectives of long-term care consumers in both institutional and community settings. This section includes research in the development of instruments for measuring satisfaction among consumers (including consumers with dementia), family members, and caregivers. Another subject related to the understanding of satisfaction measures and included in this publication is an exploration of the consumer/provider relationship and its relation to the consumers' perception of care quality.

Part III offers broad, critical, and thoughtful works on the significant changes that consumer voice and choice bring to long-term care. These authors discuss the possibility for a common consumer-centered agenda across all age groups and populations receiving long-term services, the cultural and ideological factors at play in the debate about paying family caregivers, and the challenges of defining quality from the perspectives of multiple stakeholders. This section also includes a chapter that challenges us to consider situations in which consumer self-direction is not successful. One of the authors in Part III draws on personal experience and theoretical perspectives to analyze the ways in which we structure, define, stratify, and commodify work in long-term care.

Any change in social policy—particularly change that is responsive to issues of autonomy and choice in publicly funded programs such as in consumer direction, and which addresses the needs of those with serious, chronic disabilities—can be expected to evoke strong and varied reactions. More, the reactions will reflect the interests and perspectives of various stakeholders who are involved in the change. To weigh and reconcile various aspects of this policy, we need multiple angles of vision on consumer direction. Researchers need guidance on how to study and evaluate such programs; practitioners need information on how they can best fulfill their professional roles in a changing long-term care system; policy advocates and the general public need to consider the practical and also ethical issues they must face in protecting vulnerable people. In this volume, we hope to have made steps toward addressing and clarifying both the broad range of questions and the varying and sometimes opposing perspectives of stakeholders regarding consumer direction in long-term care.

REFERENCE

Infeld, D. L. (2004). *States' experiences implementing consumer-directed home and community services: Results of the 2004 Survey of State Administrators, Opinion Survey and Telephone Interviews.* Washington, DC: National Association of State Units on Aging and The National Council on the Aging.

PART I

Consumer Choice

CHAPTER ONE

Older Consumers and Decision Making:

A Look at Family Caregivers and Care Receivers

Carol J. Whitlatch

"We have a family discussion before we make any major decision about my care. I get good care from my family."
> —78-year-old woman with dementia, cared for by her 56-year-old daughter

BACKGROUND

Families play a central role in both the decision making and delivery of long-term care to the estimated 13 to 15 million Americans with adult-onset cognitive impairment (e.g., Alzheimer's disease, stroke, Parkinson's disease, traumatic brain injury; Family Caregiver Alliance, 1999). Despite the magnitude of the number of persons living with cognitive and physical impairments, we know very little about how families make decisions about everyday care. According to Kane (1995, p. 89), "In long-term care, both the older person who perceives a need for help and family members who may decide to provide care have decisions to make. One decides whether to accept care; the other, whether to give it. Each is influenced

3

by the other, sometimes by explicit advice and sometimes by influences about what is important to the other." Few studies exist that examine the types of daily care decisions that family caregivers and care receivers make, especially when cognitive impairment is involved (Young, 1994).

Loss of cognitive and functional abilities affects the individual and his or her family in profound ways. For example, balancing the needs and preferences of the impaired person with the needs and preferences of the family caregiver can be exceedingly complex. Often at great personal sacrifice, families strive to keep a loved one at home, sometimes to avoid more costly institutional care. One of the most difficult problems a family caregiver faces is making decisions for a loved one whose capacity for planning and judgment may be impaired. Often, conflicting factors must be weighed. The following questions illustrate the nature of the conflicting need between caregivers and care receivers. *Is there a potential for risk or harm to my wife or others? How do I reconcile her wish not to let anyone in the house, with my need for help with her care?* There are no simple answers to these questions. In practice, it is oftentimes difficult to separate the needs, preferences, and best interests of the person with dementia from the needs, preferences, and best interests of the family.

Family caregivers often have a limited understanding of the needs and preferences of the relatives for whom they provide care. Caregivers may have a general understanding of what is important but do not necessarily know how important certain care values and preferences are to their relatives (Feinberg & Whitlatch, 2001; Whitlatch, Feinberg, & Tucke, in press). Adding to this already stressful situation is the reality that families have very few service options that take into account, let alone enhance, the autonomy of both caregiver and care receiver. More typically, but not always, services provide some level of choice to either the caregiver OR the care receiver. The number of services that are considered *consumer directed* is slowly increasing as both consumers and providers begin to appreciate the value of consumer direction in both community-based and residential long-term care environments.

This chapter introduces the concept of consumer direction (CD) as it applies to community-based family caregivers and the persons for whom they provide care. First, the chapter provides a brief overview of the stresses associated with family caregiving and then moves to a description of the concept of CD and the issues surrounding its development and utility within community-based programs for caregivers and care receivers. Next, the issues surrounding the implementation of consumer-directed care are discussed including family decision making when cognitive impairment is involved, the emergence of *person-centered care*, and the challenges of implementing consumer-directed programs that simultaneously serve both the caregiver and the care receiver. Third, the question is posed and discussed: *do all caregivers and care receivers want consumer-directed options?* Fourth, a brief description is given of a study that examines the care values and preferences of care receivers and whether their caregivers understand these values and preferences. The chapter ends with a discussion of the key issues to consider when designing and implementing consumer-directed programs for caregivers and care receivers.

RESEARCH ON CONSUMER DIRECTION FOR BOTH THE CAREGIVER AND CARE RECEIVER

"The hardest thing is the dependence of my parents on me. Their expectations are way too high, too much for one person. I have no time for my own life."
— 54-year-old daughter caring for her 83-year-old mother with memory problems

More and more families are facing the economic and emotional costs of providing long-term care. At the same time people with cognitive and physical disabilities are making strides toward greater autonomy through consumer-directed care. The concept of CD in home and community care is based on the key elements of choice, control, autonomy, and the philosophy that informed consumers make choices about the services they receive (National Council on the Aging, 1996). Consumer direction implies that consumers prefer to make decisions about their service needs and are able to take a more active role in managing their own services. This trend in CD is an outgrowth of the Independent Living Movement, which began in the 1970s primarily with younger adults with physical disabilities (DeJong, Batavia, & McKnew, 1992; Simon-Rusinowitz & Hofland, 1993). More recent initiatives have been successful in bridging the aging and disability communities (National Council on the Aging).

Consumer direction implies that the consumer should be presumed competent to make choices. Yet, "the presumption of competence also means that a consumer's decision to delegate responsibility for directing certain aspects of service provision to other persons can be a consumer-directed choice, in the right circumstances: for example, where a person with cognitive impairment has a family member acting as a consumer on his or her behalf" (National Council on the Aging, 1996, p. 7). Thus the notion of who is the *consumer* in long-term care is an important policy and practice issue for those designing and testing long-term care service delivery systems and interventions for persons with cognitive impairment and their informal caregivers.

In recent years, research on health care preferences, decision making, and CD has expanded in a variety of directions. Past research on CD has focused largely on end-of-life medical care in acute settings. Preferences for and decisions about do not resuscitate orders or naming a health care proxy make up the majority of this research. In contrast, few studies have examined day-to-day care preferences and decision making. Yet, some of the most difficult decisions and conflicts for persons with cognitive and/or physical impairment and their families arise in everyday long-term care at home and in community-based settings. Deciding when to bathe, what to wear, whether to purchase and use support services (e.g., in-home care or adult day services), or when to accept care from family members are examples of difficult everyday care decisions that families must make. Tremendous family conflict can occur as the care receiver progressively declines in his or her ability to carry out such daily activities as managing money, driving, or cooking. For persons with cognitive impairment, decisions and preferences about everyday care become increasingly difficult to communicate as their disease progresses and their cognitive and functional abilities deteriorate.

Questions about the family's role in home- and community-based care are complex when the person being cared for has cognitive impairment because, frequently, the family becomes both the *decision maker* and the *service provider*. According to Kapp (1996), empowering the person with cognitive impairment often means empowering his or her family support system. Past research suggests that most—but not all—adults want a family member to make health care decisions for them if they are not able to make decisions themselves (High, 1988; Louis Harris and Associates, 1982). Some care receivers, however, have no family, whereas others have families who are unable or unwilling to assume the decision-making role (Feinberg & Whitlatch, 1998). Nevertheless, few care receivers make decisions entirely without the assistance of others. It is important to understand the various roles of family members and other informal caregivers in the decision-making process when a relative has physical and/or cognitive impairments (Feasley, 1996). Thus, if consumer-directed services are to be successful, it is necessary that the providers of the services recognize the interdependence of the caregiver and care receiver.

Although very few research studies have examined the views and care preferences of persons with dementia, there are a growing number of studies that emphasize the importance of control, autonomy, self-care, and consumer-directed services (Eustis, 2000). The absence of the care receiver's perspective has led to a lack of representation of their needs in the selection of care strategies (Cohen, 1991). One reason for this oversight is that researchers have only recently begun to recognize and include persons with cognitive impairment as *legitimate contributors* in the research process (Cotrell & Schulz, 1993). As Woods (1999, p. 36) has noted, "there has been the assumption that people with dementia are unable to communicate in a meaningful way, invalidating their participation in decision making about their own situation as well as rendering their lived experience and their perspective as being impossible to research." According to Stewart, Sherbourne, and Brod (1996), subjective assessment in cognitively impaired populations has been ignored because of the presumed logistical and methodological issues, specifically regarding comprehension and reliability. Sadly, researchers and practitioners often wrongly assume that persons with cognitive impairment are unable to make care decisions for themselves. As a result, there are very few model consumer-directed programs that recognize the impaired adult's voice in decision making.

Recently, however, in both research and practice, there has been a move to understand the preferences and experiences of persons with dementia (Downs, 1997; Kitwood & Benson, 1995; Woods, 1999). The majority of the literature on the emergence of the person in dementia research is qualitative in design. Downs (1997) outlines three areas that have been studied: (1) the individual's sense of self, (2) perspectives of persons with dementia, and (3) a person's rights. In terms of sense of self, a growing body of research suggests that people with dementia retain a sense of self, despite cognitive impairment, into the late stages of the illness (Downs; Kitwood, 1997; Woods, 1999). Further evidence that persons with dementia are able to report on their situation comes from the growing number of support groups and other services developed specifically for persons with early-stage dementia (Brod, Stewart, Sands, & Walton, 1999; Yale, 1999). Downs (p. 605) notes that although more attention has recently been paid to the perspectives of persons with dementia, there is a "clear bias towards eliciting views from people in the early stages." Last, there is a growing trend acknowledging the rights of people with dementia (Downs). A gap still exists, however, in exploring the person's values, preferences, and decision making for daily care situations.

To date, no valid, standardized method exists to determine decisional capacity (Gerety, Chiodo, Kanten, Tuley, & Cornell, 1993; Kapp & Mossman, 1996). In home- and community-based care, capacity is oftentimes best assessed on a decision-specific basis, where some persons with cognitive impairment may have decisional capacity in some respects but lack capacity in others. For example, Mrs. M. may be able to decide who should make health care decisions for her if she is no longer able, but not competent enough to shop for groceries. Because of the intellectual impairment that characterizes most dementing illnesses, the capacity to make decisions about daily activities is often compromised (Zarit & Goodman, 1990). When cognitive impairment is mild, questions may arise about the care receiver's ability to perform certain activities (e.g., to continue working or handle financial affairs). If cognitive functioning further deteriorates, care receivers are faced with decisions about daily life activities that may jeopardize the safety of both the person with cognitive impairment and others (e.g., driving and cooking; Zarit & Goodman). In the advanced stage of dementia, for example, language deficits limit the individual's ability to communicate. Unless the care receiver had previously expressed preferences for everyday care, it is nearly impossible to know what the individual wants and needs (Cotrell & Schulz, 1993).

Although it appears that care receivers with mild to moderate cognitive impairments are able to voice their preferences and make informed decisions about a variety of care-related issues (Brod et al., 1999; Cohen & Eisdorfer, 1986; Gerety et al., 1993; Logsdon & Teri, 1996; McHorney, 1996; Parmlee, Lawton, & Katz, 1989; Sansone, Schmitt, & Nichols, 1996), the impact of this consumer-driven movement on family caregivers is unknown. Does empowering the care receiver lead to a disempowered caregiver? Is care receiver and caregiver empowerment mutually exclusive? Preliminary evidence suggests that increased involvement in decision making by care receivers is associated with higher levels of caregiver depression (Whitlatch, 1999). To illustrate, a daughter caring for her mildly demented father may find that his involvement in decision making is counter to her own best interests. She may wish to make all decisions herself, for example, preferring for her father to remain safe at home with paid assistance. The father might prefer to be alone during the day and check in with his daughter hourly by telephone. When do his rights to consumer-directed care supercede her rights and vice versa? Does his previously voiced preference to remain at home rather than be placed in a facility override her preference if his home care becomes too much for her? Often, one's assessment of need changes according to circumstances making it particularly difficult both to project future change in circumstance and to anticipate evolving preferences and options to those changes (Hibbard, Slovic, & Jewett, 1997). Again, there are no easy answers to these very real questions and dilemmas.

DO CAREGIVERS AND CARE RECEIVERS WANT CONSUMER-DIRECTED OPTIONS?

"I have no personal or down time. It is affecting my health. If I had some more personal time, I could do a better job of caregiving."
—66-year-old wife caring for her 65-year-old husband with memory problems

It is widely assumed that family caregivers and care receivers prefer service delivery options that include consumer-directed models. This assumption is a product of the trend toward increased self-determination and consumer direction. However, there are a number of factors that may be linked to a person's interest in receiving consumer-directed services. Research suggests that cost plays a central role in determining access to and interest in receiving care, and in the type and duration of care received (Advisory Panel on Alzheimer's Disease, 1992; Wilson, 1995). But how do costs influence family caregiver and care receiver preferences for and decisions about the use of consumer-directed home and community-based care? Results of recent research on consumer choice for family caregivers indicate that the direct pay (i.e., consumer-directed) model of in-home respite is the preferred mode of service delivery (Feinberg & Whitlatch, 1998). Caregivers who preferred the consumer-directed option were more likely to be employed outside the home and more likely to be of an ethnic minority group. Moreover, the consumer-directed model was more cost effective than the agency-based respite care model (Feinberg & Whitlatch). Specifically, caregivers who used the consumer-directed option received more hours of respite care than caregivers who used agency-based respite. In addition, compared to agency-based respite, the direct-pay option was shown to be significantly less costly per hour of service. On the other hand, results also suggested that caregivers in both groups (i.e., direct-pay and agency-based users) valued safety concerns and good, reliable, and trustworthy help over cost issues and amount of care. Thus, cost of care is just one of many critical factors that families consider when they are choosing the care options that best fit their needs.

Autonomy, choice, and consumer-directed options are important to community dwelling consumers as well as to those living in residential settings. Findings from a study of nearly 300 long-term care receivers suggest that consumers had clear preferences for both initial and continued control over personal decision making (Salmon & Polivka, 2000). When given three options for how care should be provided, one-third (34%) of home care consumers preferred consumer-directed options, 13% preferred a traditional agency model, and the remaining showed no preference or did not like any of the three models (Salmon & Polivka). Similarly, Simon-Rusinowitz and colleagues (1997; Simon-Rusinowitz, Bochniak, Mahoney, Marks, & Hecht, 2000) suggest that a sizable number of the older consumers they interviewed were interested in consumer-directed options.

Yet, not all older adults prefer consumer-directed program options. This is true for persons regardless of ethnicity, age, and cognitive ability. Research that examined elder judgments to questions regarding community long-term care showed significant racial and ethnic group differences regarding desire for and satisfaction with control over the amount, type, and manner of care (Sciegaj, 2001). African American, Latino, and White elders who were receiving community-based case management services reported a preference for traditional models of care rather than more consumer-directed models (e.g., cash and counseling). Chinese elders were equally likely to prefer a Social Health Maintenance Organization (SHMO) model (47%) or a traditional model (50%) to a more consumer-directed model of community care (Sciegaj). In this case, the elders' preference for the SHMO and traditional models may be accounted for by their having received care from culturally appropriate care agencies (Sciegaj). More recently, Sciegaj, Capitman, and Kyriacou (2004) report that elders, regardless of racial and ethnic background, who desire control over in-home care workers are less likely to select a traditional case management service option. The findings of these studies suggest that community long-term care judgments are the result of a complex configuration of racial, ethnic, and gender differences in social experiences that have not been captured in previous studies.

In general, few studies examine how families make decisions about everyday and long-term care. Central to this issue is the question of whether caregivers understand their relatives' care values and preferences. We next move to a discussion of preliminary findings from one of the first studies to examine care receiver's values and preferences for care from the perspective of both caregivers and care receivers.

CAREGIVER AND CARE RECEIVER VALUES AND PREFERENCES FOR CARE

"I need a break, some time to get away with assurance that mother is in safe hands."
> —50-year-old daughter caring for her 71-year-old mother

Following the work of Ogletree (1995), Degenholtz, Kane, and Kivnick (1997, p. 768) define *"values* as broad beliefs about features in the everyday world to which people attach importance, and *preferences* as more specific choices that flow from values." Drawing on this definition, we developed the *Values and Preferences Scale* from previous work with cognitively intact samples (Degenholtz et al.; Kane & Degenholtz, 1997; McCullough, Wilson, Teasdale, Kolpakchi, & Skelly, 1993). Exploratory factor analyses of the caregivers' responses indicated that the 37 items of values and preferences in everyday care that the care receiver felt were "very important," "somewhat important," or "not at all important" could be collapsed into four conceptual domains:

1. Self identity/Environment (10 items, alpha = .71)
2. Autonomy (9 items, alpha = .80)
3. Burden (4 items, alpha = .70)
4. Family and social network (14 items, alpha = .79).

Table 1.1 Top Seven Values and Preferences Scale Items for Care Receivers (CRs) and Caregivers (CGs)

	CR	Mean	CG	Mean
Be safe from crime	1	2.91	4	2.87
Have a comfortable place to live	2	2.90	3	2.90
Feel safe in home, even if it restricts activities	3	2.89	2	2.91
Maintain dignity	4	2.81	1	2.92
Be in touch with others in case of emergency	5	2.78	8	2.66
Have reliable help	6	2.75	5	2.75
Have caregiver be the one to help out	7	2.74	6	2.73
Not live in a nursing home	13	2.53	7	2.69

The sample for which the following results are drawn consisted of 60 African American family caregiver–care receiver dyads from northeast Ohio. To be eligible for the study, African American older adults had to (1) have one or more chronic health conditions (e.g., diabetes and high blood pressure), (2) have symptoms of memory problems or an adult-onset brain disease or disorder (e.g., Alzheimer's disease, stroke, and Parkinson's disease), (3) be living at home rather than an institutional setting, and (4) be mildly to moderately cognitively impaired (scores between 13 and 26, on the Folstein Mini-Mental State Exam). Caregivers had to be the primary nonpaid caregiver for the cognitively impaired adult.

Table 1.1 lists the seven most important Values and Preferences items for care receivers and caregivers. For care receivers, the top seven items were "Be safe from crime" (2.91), "Have a comfortable place to live" (2.90), "Feel safe in home, even if it restricts activities" (2.89), "Maintain dignity" (2.81), "Be in touch with others in case of emergency" (2.78), "Have reliable help" (2.75), and "Have caregiver be the one to help out" (2.74). For caregivers, the top seven items were, "Maintain dignity" (2.92), "Feel safe in home, even if it restricts activities" (2.91), "Have a comfortable place to live" (2.90), "Be safe from crime" (2.87), "Have reliable help" (2.75), "Have caregiver be the one to help out" (2.73), and "Not live in a nursing home" (2.69). At the group level, item means for the care receivers and caregivers were often slightly different. Yet, none of the item means for the seven highest ranked items were significantly different (see Table 1.1).

Next, responses of care receivers were compared to the responses of caregivers on each of the 37 items in the Values and Preferences scale. T-tests determined whether there was congruence or agreement between care receivers and caregivers. In other words, if there were significant

Table 1.2 Care Receiver and Caregiver Values and Preferences Item Means and Significant t-values

	Care Receiver	Caregiver Mean	t-value
Autonomy			
Use services only covered by insurance	2.18	1.71	−3.531**
Have say in excluding family or friends from helping	2.05	2.39	3.705**
Burden			
Have money to leave to family	2.00	1.64	−2.685*
Caregiver not put life on hold	2.65	2.40	−2.037*
Self-identity/environment			
Do things for self	2.68	2.38	−2.562*
Have something to do	2.50	2.10	−3.584**
Use services can pay for by self	2.25	1.75	−3.521**
Family/social network			
Do things with other people	2.39	2.12	−2.376*
Maintain continuity with the past	2.17	2.44	2.167*

*p < .05.
**p < .01.

differences in how important the caregivers thought the item was to the care receiver and how important the item actually was to the care receiver, the item was considered incongruent. Significant differences were found for 9 of the 37 items (see Table 1.2). Typically when there were significant differences, the care receiver placed greater importance on the item than the caregiver thought they did. For example, care receivers felt the item "Caregiver not put life on hold" from the Burden subscale was significantly more important than caregivers felt it was to care receivers (2.65 vs. 2.40, $p < .05$). One exception to this trend is that caregivers placed greater importance on their relative's "Maintaining continuity with the past" (2.17 vs. 2.40, $p < .05$). No items from the Environment domain were found to be significantly different.

The sample was next divided by kin group (dyads with spouse caregivers, $N = 35$ and dyads with adult child caregivers, $N = 16$) and t-tests were again performed between caregiver and care receiver responses for each group. Dyads with spouse caregivers yielded significantly different care receiver and caregiver answers on 10 of the 37 items. The dyads with adult children caregivers had significantly different answers on 12 of the 37 items. As with the sample as a whole, when there were significant differences, the care receivers typically placed greater importance on the item than the caregivers thought they did. One exception to this trend appeared on one item in the dyads with spouse caregivers. Here, the spouse caregivers believed the care receivers placed more importance on "Maintain dignity" than care receivers actually did.

Finally, adult child caregivers' responses were compared to spouse caregivers' responses for each item in the *Values and Preferences Scale*. Significant differences between adult child caregivers and spouse caregivers were found for only four items, "Live in own home" (adult child mean = 2.50, spouse mean = 2.91, $t = -2.69$, $p = .010$), "Be in touch with others in case of emergency" (adult child mean = 1.81, spouse mean = 2.29, $t = -2.17$, $p = .035$), and "Have time to self" (adult child mean = 2.44, spouse mean = 1.97, $t = 2.49$, $p = .016$), and "Have caregiver be the one to help out" (adult child mean = 2.63, spouse mean = 2.94, $t = -2.67$, $p = .010$). There were no significant differences between the responses of care receivers with adult child caregivers and care receivers with spouse caregivers.

The findings from this study indicate that family caregivers have a fairly accurate view of the care values and preferences that are important to their relatives. However, caregivers are less accurate in their perceptions of *how* important certain values are to their relatives. Typically, when there is a misunderstanding, the caregiver underestimates the importance of a specific value. The exception, "Maintain continuity with the past," may reflect the caregiver's own difficulty in letting go of their relative and the relationship they once had together. In general, however, caregivers have a sense of what is important, but not how important certain values and preferences are to their relatives.

CAN CONSUMER DIRECTION BE ACHIEVED FOR BOTH CAREGIVERS AND CARE RECEIVERS?

"Coming to some understanding of what IS in the best interest of my mother, is the hardest part."
> —48-year-old daughter caring for her mother who has Alzheimer's disease

Autonomy, control, and self-determination are important to most everyone regardless of age or physical or cognitive ability. Consumer direction is much more than having the freedom to choose one's worker or assistant (Scala & Nerney, 2000). One of the main principles of CD is that informed consumers make decisions about their care or, in the case of family caregiving, the care of their relatives. In most instances, family caregivers are able to make decisions about the care of their impaired relatives. But can persons with cognitive impairments make decisions and voice their own preferences? Mounting evidence suggests that persons with mild to moderate levels of cognitive impairment are able to answer questions with a high degree of reliability and accuracy. These mild to moderately impaired care receivers possess sufficient capacity to state specific preferences, provide valid responses to questions about their demographics and their own involvement in everyday living, make care-related decisions, and express values and wishes regarding care they are receiving or would need in the future (Feinberg & Whitlatch, 2001). This research suggests that it may be useful for families and practitioners to incorporate a structured values assessment as part of interventions to improve education and enhance communication between care receivers and family caregivers around the issues of daily-care preferences.

Drawing upon these findings, Whitlatch and Zarit (2003, November) are designing and evaluating an intervention to help families (i.e., the caregiver and care receiver) who are experiencing the early stages of dementia or other cognitive impairment. The goals of this intervention study, funded by the National Family Caregiver Support Program, are to develop positive communication patterns between the caregiver and the care receiver; increase knowledge and understanding of available services, preferences for care, and care values; and increase the care receiver's active participation in his or her care plan. In turn, caregivers and care receivers are expected to experience improved well-being, self-esteem, and an increased sense of self-efficacy in managing the consequences of cognitive impairment. This dyadic intervention is one of the first to embrace the concepts of consumer direction for both the caregiver and the care receiver.

The number of consumer-directed programs and interventions that serve caregivers and care receivers is slowly increasing. The range and scope of these programs vary greatly according to funding source, financial resources, population served, and organizational capacity. As more consumer-directed programs are developed and implemented, it is important to remember a few key issues:

1. Not all consumers want or will use consumer-driven service options.
2. Empowering the caregiver can have a tremendous impact, either negative or positive, on the care receiver.
3. Empowering the care receiver can have a tremendous impact, either negative or positive, on the caregiver.
4. No single consumer-directed model will be useful in all settings, thus flexible designs in consumer-directed care are crucial.
5. Consumer-directed programs must be thoroughly evaluated, modified, and re-evaluated if they are to be efficient and effective.

6. The results of program evaluations must be disseminated widely to ensure the continuation and replication of effective consumer-directed programs.

Consideration of these six issues is vital to the success and continuation of consumer-directed programs. Public policies that acknowledge persons with cognitive impairment *and* family caregivers as legitimate *consumers* of long-term care will provide additional support to the development of effective and innovative consumer-directed services. Moreover, increased understanding of the preferences of the person with cognitive or physical impairment and the needs of the family caregiver will improve the decision-making process, lead to more informed decisions, and reduce the strain on family caregivers and associated health costs. It is, after all, family caregivers, who are today and will continue to be in the foreseeable future, the major providers of long-term care.

ACKNOWLEDGMENTS

This manuscript was supported in part by Contract 282-98-0016, Task Order 26, from the Administration on Aging, Department of Health and Human Services, Washington, DC 20201. Points of view and considerations expressed in this manuscript are those of the author and do not necessarily represent official Administration on Aging policy. The research presented was supported by the Retirement Research Foundation, the Robert Wood Johnson Foundation, the AARP Andrus Foundation, and the National Institute on Aging P50 AG-08012-16.

REFERENCES

Advisory Panel on Alzheimer's Disease. (1992). *Third report of the advisory panel on Alzheimer's disease, 1991*. DHHS Pub. No. (ADM)92-1917. Washington, DC: Superintendent of Documents, U.S. Government Printing Office.

Brod, M., Stewart, A. L., Sands, L., & Walton, P. (1999). Conceptualization and measurement of quality of life in dementia: The dementia quality of life instrument (DQOL). *The Gerontologist, 39*, 25–35.

Cohen, D. (1991). The subjective experience of Alzheimer's disease. The anatomy of an illness as perceived by patients and families. *American Journal of Alzheimer's Care and Related Disorders and Research, 6*, 6–11.

Cohen, D., & Eisdorfer, C. (1986). *The loss of self*. New York: Norton.

Cotrell, V., & Schulz, R. (1993). The perspective of the patient with Alzheimer's disease: A neglected dimension of dementia research. *The Gerontologist, 33*, 205–211.

Degenholtz, H., Kane, R. A., & Kivnick, H. Q. (1997). Care-related preferences and values of elderly community-based long term care consumers: Can care managers learn what's important to clients? *The Gerontologist, 37,* 767–776.

DeJong, G., Batavia, A. I., & McKnew, L. B. (1992). The independent living model of personal assistance in national long-term care policy. *Generations, 16,* 89–95.

Downs, M. (1997). Progress report: The emergence of the person in dementia research. *Aging and Society, 17,* 597–604.

Eustis, N. (2000). Consumer-directed long-term care services: Evolving perspectives and alliances. *Generations, 24*(3), 10–15.

Family Caregiver Alliance. (1999). *Prevalence of the major causes of adult-onset brain impairment in the United States.* San Francisco, CA: Family Caregiver Alliance.

Feasely, J. C. (1996). *Health outcomes for older people: Questions for the coming decade.* Washington, DC: National Academy Press.

Feinberg, L. F., & Whitlatch, C. J. (1998). Family caregivers and in-home respite options: The consumer-directed versus agency-based experience. *Journal of Gerontological Social Work, 30*(3), 9–28.

Feinberg, L. F., & Whitlatch, C. J. (2001). Are persons with cognitive impairment able to state consistent choices? *The Gerontologist, 41,* 374–362.

Gerety, M. B., Chiodo, L. K., Kanten, D. N., Tuley, M. R., & Cornell, J. E. (1993). Medical treatment preferences of nursing home residents: Relationship to function and concordance with surrogate decision makers. *Journal of the American Geriatrics Society, 41,* 953–960.

Hibbard, J. H., Slovic, P. & Jewett, J. J. (1997). Informing consumer decisions in health care: Implications from decision-making research. *Milbank Quarterly, 75,* 395–414.

High, D. M. (1988). All in the family: Extended autonomy and expectations in surrogate health care decision making. *The Gerontologist,* 28(Suppl.), 46–51.

Kane, R. (1995). Decision making, care plans and life plans. In L. B. McCullough & N. L. Wilson (Eds.), *Long term care decisions: Ethical and conceptual dimensions.* Baltimore, MD: The Johns Hopkins Press.

Kane, R., & Degenholtz, H. (1997). Assessing values and preferences: Should we, can we? *Generations, 21,* 19–21.

Kapp, M. B. (1996). Enhancing autonomy and choice in selecting and directing long-term care services. *The Elder Law Journal, 4,* 55–97.

Kapp, M. B., & Mossman, D. (1996). Measuring decisional capacity: Cautions on the construction of a capacimeter. *Psychology, Public Health and the Law, 2,* 73–95.

Kitwood, T. (1997). The experience of dementia. *Aging and Mental Health, I,* 13–22.

Kitwood, T., & Benson, S. (1995). *The new culture of dementia care.* London: Hawker Publications.

Logsdon, R., & Teri, L. (1996, November). *Assessment of quality of life, pleasant events, and depression in Alzheimer's disease outpatients.* Paper presented at the annual meeting of the Gerontological Society of America, Washington, DC.

Louis Harris and Associates. (1982). Views of informed consent and decision-making: Parallel surveys of physicians and the public. In President's Commission for the Study of Ethical Problems in Medicine and Biomedical and Behavioral Research. *Making health care decisions: A report on the ethical and legal implications of informed consent in the patient practitioner relationship*. Washington, DC: U.S. Government Printing Office.

McCullough, L. B., Wilson, N. L., Teasdale, T. T., Kolpakchi, A. L., & Skelly, J. R. (1993). Mapping personal, familial and professional values in long term care decisions. *The Gerontologist, 33*, 324–332.

McHorney, C. A. (1996). Measuring and monitoring general health status in elderly persons: Practical and methodological issues in using the SF-36 Health Survey. *The Gerontologist, 36*, 571–583.

National Council on the Aging. (1996, July). *Principles of consumer-directed home and community-based services*. Washington, DC: National Institute on Consumer-Directed Long Term Care Services, National Council on the Aging.

Ogletree, T. W. (1995). Values and valuation. In W. T. Reich (Ed.), *Encyclopedia of bioethics: Revised edition* (Vol. 5, pp. 2515–2520), New York: MacMillan.

Parmlee, P. A., Lawton, M. P., & Katz, I. R. (1989). Psychometric properties of the Geriatric Depression Scale among the institutionalized aged. *Psychological Assessment, 1*, 331–338.

Salmon, J.R., & Polivka, L. (2000). Study shows link between control and consumer satisfaction. *Consumer Choice News, 4*(4), 4, 6, 8.

Sansone, P., Schmitt, R. L., & Nichols, J. N. (1996). *The right to choose: Capacity study of demented residents in nursing homes*. New York, NY: Frances Schervier Home and Hospital.

Scala, M.A., & Nerney, T. (2000). People first: The consumers in consumer direction. *Generations, 24(3)*, 55–59.

Sciegaj, M. (2001) Elder preferences for consumer direction. Paper presented at Consumer Voice and Choice, Scripps Gerontology Center, Fourth Conference on Long-Term Care. October 18, 2001, Columbus Ohio.

Sciegaj, M., Capitman, J.A., & Kyriacou, C.K. (2004). Consumer-directed community care: Race/ethnicity and individual differences in preferences for control. *The Gerontologist, 44*(4), 489–499.

Simon-Rusinowitz, L., Bochniak, A. M., Mahoney, K. J., Marks, L. N., & Hecht, D. (2000). Implementation issues for consumer-directed programs: A survey of policy experts. *Generations, 24*(3), 34–40.

Simon-Rusinowitz, L., & Hofland, B. F. (1993). Adopting a disability approach to home care services for older adults. *The Gerontologist, 33*, 159–167.

Simon-Rusinowitz, L., Mahoney, K., Desmond, S., Shoop, D., Squillace, M., & Fay, R. (1997). Determining consumer preferences for a cash option: Arkansas survey results. *Health Care Financing Review, 19*(2), 87.

Stewart, A., Sherbourne, C., & Brod, M. (1996). Measuring health-related quality of life in older and demented populations. In B. Spilker (Ed.), *Quality of life and pharmaeconomics in clinical trials: Second edition* (pp. 819–829). Philadelphia: Lippincott-Rasen.

Whitlatch, C. J. (1999, November). The impact of culture on healthcare decision-making for caregiving families. In E. E. MaloneBeach & C. J. Whitlatch (Organizers). *Culture and caregiving in African American families.* Symposium conducted at the Annual Meeting of the Gerontological Society of America, San Francisco.

Whitlatch, C. J., Feinberg, L. F., & Tucke, S. T. (in press). Accuracy and consistency of responses from persons with dementia. *Dementia: The International Journal of Social Research and Practice.*

Whitlatch, C. J., & Zarit, S. (2003, November). *Research and interventions with family caregivers and persons with dementia: Respecting both voices.* Symposium presented at the Annual Meeting of the Gerontological Society of America, San Diego, CA.

Wilson, N. L. (1995). Long-term care in the United States: An overview of the current system. In L. B. McCullough and N. L. Wilson (Eds.), *Long-term care decisions: Ethical and conceptual dimensions.* Baltimore: The Johns Hopkins University Press.

Woods, B. (1999). The person in dementia care. *Generations, 23,* 35–39.

Yale, R. (1999). Support groups and other services for individuals with early-stage Alzheimer's disease. *Generations, 23,* 57–61.

Young, R. (1994). Elders, families and illness. *Journal of Aging Studies, 8,* 115.

Zarit, S. H., & Goodman, C. R. (1990). Decision making and dementia. *The American Journal of Alzheimer's Care and Related Disorders and Research,* September–October, 22–28.

RECOMMENDED RESOURCES ON CONSUMER DIRECTION

National Council on the Aging. (1996, July). *Principles of consumer-directed home and community-based services.* Washington, DC: National Institute on Consumer-Directed Long Term Care Services, National Council on the Aging.

The entire issue of the journal *Generations (Volume 24, no. 3, Fall 2000)* is devoted to a variety of topics related to consumer direction. This volume is titled "Consumer Direction in Long-Term Care" and is a publication of the American Society on Aging, 833 Market Street, San Francisco CA 94103-1824, www.asaging.org.

For further information on the Cash and Counseling Demonstration and Evaluation contact the University of Maryland Center on Aging, www.inform.umd.edu/aging.

Doty, P., Kasper, J., & Litvak, S. (1996). Consumer directed models of personal care: Lessons from Medicaid. *The Milbank Quarterly, 74,* 377–409.

Commonwealth Fund Commission on Elderly Living Alone. (1991). *The impor-
    tance of choice in Medicaid home care programs: Maryland, Michigan, and
    Texas.* New York: Louis Harris and Associates.
For further information on California's statewide system of consumer directed
    Caregiver Resource Centers contact Lynn Friss Feinberg, Deputy Direc-
    tor, National Center on Caregiving, Family Caregiver Alliance, 690 Market
    Street, Suite 600, San Francisco, CA 94108, www.caregiver.org.

CHAPTER TWO

Choice and the Institutionalized Elderly

Susan C. Reinhard
Sandra Howell White
Winifred Quinn

BACKGROUND

One of the hallmarks of American life is the ability to choose how one lives it. Until recently, this basic value did not get much attention in the long-term care (LTC) field. Too often, older adults and persons with disabilities who have difficulty managing the tasks of daily living and the challenges of chronic health conditions have had little choice or help in making decisions about long-term care. In particular, the forces driving frail elders into institutional care have been well documented (Kane, Kane, & Ladd, 1998). Once placed in a nursing home, people often find it difficult to return home or to another community-based setting. The prevailing assumption is that the decision to enter a nursing home is generally a final decision. The idea that the older adult's condition might improve, or that there may be other alternatives outside of a nursing home, is a foreign concept to many. Even some advocates for the elderly believe a nursing home is the safest place for those who have crossed a particular physical or cognitive threshold. Crossing back seems unthinkable. Concerted effort is needed to change this thinking.

INTRODUCTION

In 1998, New Jersey developed the Community Choice Counseling (CCC) initiative to help institutionalized older adults and younger persons with

disabilities find more options to return to their communities. The process of developing this program and the early evaluation findings provide
lessons for other state policymakers, community leaders, and advocates.
Researchers at Rutgers Center for State Health Policy evaluated the CCC
program at the request of the New Jersey Department of Health and Senior Services (NJDHSS). This chapter illustrates the research findings and
based on those findings provides suggestions for implementing further
initiatives.

POLICY DEVELOPMENT: CREATING CHOICES

During the 1990s, New Jersey's health and aging policy community
developed consensus that the state needed to develop more LTC alternatives for its frail older adults (NJDHSS, 1991). Through a process of
public hearings, consumers, providers, and policymakers concurred that
the state should make a determined effort to create more LTC options.
In 1995, state officials designed a conceptual framework to guide that
work.

Adapted from Oregon, this model is a series of concentric circles representing a variety of services for older adults (see Figure 2.1). Institutional
(nursing home) care is in the center with increasingly more homelike services and health-promotion programs in circles away from the center. The
outermost circles represent home- and community-based services, such as
day care and meals on wheels, and the final circle represents programs
that promote wellness. The goal of this model is to help people "stick"
to the outer circles, where they most often prefer to be, and where more
choice and autonomy are possible. An important feature of this model
is that people can move in and out of these various circles—movement
should not be thought of as ultimately unidirectional or linear. In this
model people can move from any circle to another and back again, and
to any other circle between as their changing circumstances require and
allow, and just as importantly as their preferences dictate.

Many policy changes are needed to actualize this conceptual model
and enhance consumer choice. For the past several years, New Jersey has
been working on several initiatives to promote independence, dignity, and
choice for older adults and persons with disabilities.

The first initiative started in 1996 with the creation of a locally
based information and assistance system so older adults and their families
could learn about their options. Known as New Jersey Easy Access Single
Entry (NJEASE), the goal was to consolidate all services at the local level
through the use of a toll-free number allowing consumers to easily access

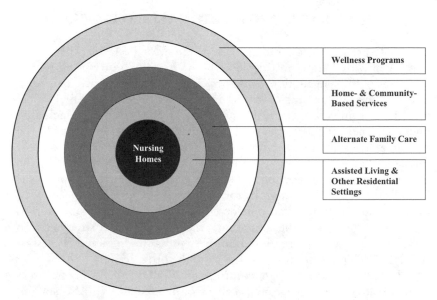

Wellness Programs

Home- & Community-Based Services

Alternate Family Care

Assisted Living & Other Residential Settings

Nursing Homes

Figure 2.1   The New Jersey Department of Health and Senior Service's Model for Promoting Independence.

information to make informed choices about LTC services (Reinhard & Scala, 2001).

At the same time, consolidation of all senior services at the state level led to the creation of the NJDHSS. This consolidation brought together Medicaid funding for nursing homes and home- and community-based waivers serving older adults, regulatory development of the new options like assisted living and alternate family care, quality oversight of these services, the aging network served by the state unit on aging, and health promotion services. With one state agency responsible for all of the funding, licensing, and inspection of all LTC services, the power to redesign that system was enhanced. Creating more options for long-term care was a prerequisite for this redesign. In 1996, New Jersey was considered "below average" in the proportion of all LTC expenditures that went to home- and community-based care—with a ranking of 21 among the states (Ladd, 1999). After considerable program development, in 1999 the state budgeted $60 million in state and federal dollars to develop more consumer-directed home care options, and more respite care for family caregivers (Reinhard & Fahey, 2003). Known collectively as the "Senior Initiatives," this funding expanded a pilot program started in 1998 to make sure older adults in nursing homes were also able to find out about these choices. That program was named Community Choice Counseling or CCC.

CHOICES FOR INSTITUTIONALIZED ELDERS

The CCC program grew out of a pilot initiative in 1998. This initiative began with 2 state staff persons, both registered nurses, and within 4 months of implementation, 300 nursing home residents were helped to return to their homes and communities. Telephone follow-up of 10% of these former nursing home residents found positive outcomes, including high consumer satisfaction, few re-hospitalizations, and low costs to the consumer and state for community placement. Staff found that some of these older adults and persons with disabilities had "gotten stuck" in the nursing home setting. For some, the admission to the nursing home was intended to be for a few months for recovery from an illness or an accident. Without help from an outside contact who could provide help to get the resident back to the community, their length of stay stretched into 6 months, a year, or more. Based on these initial findings and successes, NJDHSS decided to continue and expand the program.

To prepare for the expanded program, NJDHSS senior officials met with the directors of the county offices on aging, the NJEASE staff in each county, and nursing home industry leaders to discuss the goals of the program and to plan the deployment of 40 nurses and social workers to counsel selected nursing home residents. The Medicaid rules in New Jersey include requirements for prescreening assessment of all persons entering a nursing home who are either currently Medicaid beneficiaries or likely to become financially eligible for Medicaid within 6 months of admission to a nursing home. Because most people fall into the latter category, New Jersey's rules already offer the opportunity for screening and counseling for the majority of people entering a nursing home. Additional staffing, training, and LTC service alternatives were the fundamental elements needed to make CCC a viable initiative.

The CCC protocol calls for trained state-employed staff to conduct a full needs assessment and identify the applicant into one of three categories: likely to be a long-term nursing home admission, able to receive services in the community through a Medicaid waiver program or some other service, or potentially able to return to the community after a re-evaluation within 6 months. The CCC staff started by focusing on the last two groups, but was given the discretion to reassess anyone who requested counseling or appeared to be appropriate for counseling. These staff members needed training and opportunities to rethink their traditional role as "Medicaid screeners" as they became "community choice counselors." In addition, state nursing home survey staff was trained to identify nursing home residents who might benefit from CCC.

Through regional meetings with the CCC staff, senior NJDHSS officials sought to contend with the issues staff experienced in redefining their roles. Some CCC staff members reported initial resistance from nursing home staff. In more than one case, nursing home discharge planners stated that they feared dismissal from their jobs if they cooperated with the community choice counselors (Lagnado, 2001). Many counselors felt they needed continually updated information about community resources and materials to help them explain various nursing home alternatives. A grant from the Centers for Medicare and Medicaid Services (CMS) helped fund the development of those materials.

PROGRAM EVALUATION

NJDHSS contracted with the Rutgers Center for State Health Policy (CSHP) in 1999 to design and implement an objective, formative program evaluation. This chapter summarizes the findings from the first four months of the evaluation, from January 1 through April 30, 2000, with a focus on three areas: the clients' current living situation (8 to 10 weeks after the transition from a nursing home—a critical period), the use of informal and formal assistance, and quality of life.

Methods

To evaluate the CCC program, CSHP used information from discharge summary forms from 688 nursing home clients that the community choice counselors helped to transition from nursing homes between January 1, 2000, and April 30, 2000, and which were provided by NJDHSS. Eight to 10 weeks after the nursing home resident was discharged, the research team contacted them to conduct a telephone survey. The 2-month post-discharge timeframe was chosen to ensure that the person had sufficient time to settle into their new setting and experience community services. The CSHP staff asked questions about how satisfied they were with their current living situation, what kind of services they were receiving from family and paid caregivers, and inquired about the quality of their life in general.

When possible, the CSHP research team interviewed the person who had been discharged from the nursing home. However, they did use a proxy when the client's mental or physical condition impeded his or her participation, or the client preferred that the proxy be interviewed. When a proxy was used, the client (if able) was asked to confirm the proxy choice. In a small number of cases, both clients and their proxies completed the interviews.

In total, 358 of the 688 former nursing home residents were interviewed (see Table 2.1). One hundred and one clients (14.6%) refused to

Table 2.1 Sample Disposition

Results	Total sampling Frame	Average Age*	Average Length of Stay (Days) in NH[1]
Surveyed	358	73.5 ($n = 259$)	85.6 ($n = 281$)
Unable to participate	44	73.6 ($n = 36$)	258.7 ($n = 40$)**
Refused	101	76.2 ($n = 86$)	139.4 ($n = 99$)**
Deceased	57	76.8 ($n = 48$)	49.1 ($n = 55$)**
Unable to reach/locate	128	68.6 ($n = 107$)	136.8 ($n = 124$)**
Total	688	73.3 ($n = 536$)	114.6 ($n = 599$)

[1] This information was not available for all clients.
*Significantly different ($p < .01$) between the groups $F = 3.5$.
**Significantly different ($p < .01$) from the average length of stay of those who participated.

participate. Another 44 people (6.4%) were unable to participate because they had a physical or mental impairment and had no one who could or would serve as a proxy respondent. CSHP was unable to locate 128 clients (18.6%). Another 57 clients (8.3%) were deceased by the time the researchers attempted to reach them. Excluding the deceased and those who were unable to participate due to physical or mental impairment, the overall response rate was 61% (358/587).

Although the average age of the former nursing home residents in this sample was 73.3, with a range of 24 to 98 (SD 14.31 years; see Table 2.1), almost 20% were younger than 65 with 12.5% between the ages of 24 and 54. Although this chapter focuses on "choice and the institutionalized elderly," the CCC program is a nursing home transition program designed to assist people of all ages.

As usually seen in nursing home populations, most respondents were female (65.8%)and not married (78%). Almost all in the sample spoke English. Regarding educational level, one-third of the clients had completed high school. One-fifth of the respondents had some high school and another one-fifth had some college.

The CCC program was designed to begin its effort with those who had been in the nursing home less than 6 months but would have been at risk of remaining there if they had not received some outside help. Therefore the research team wanted to examine the length of stay (LOS) data.

Of the 688 people discharged, the average LOS was 114.6 days, with a range of 4 to 3,388 days. For those who agreed to be interviewed, the average LOS was 85.6 days (almost 3 months—the target group), with a range of 4 to 1,600 days. For those who the researchers were unable to locate, the average LOS was 136.8 days (more than 4 months), with a range of 5 to 2,296 days. The average LOS was even longer for those who could not do the interview, 258.7 days, with a range of 4 to 2,572 days. Those who had died before the researchers attempted to contact them had an average LOS of about 50 days (with a range of 4 to 334 days). Finally, those who refused to participate in the study had an average LOS of 139.4 days (with a range of 10 to 3,388 days). Given these data, the LOS for people who the research team was able to survey was significantly shorter than that for those who researchers were not able to survey. All categories of nonrespondents had significantly different lengths of stay from respondents.

Questionnaire

The survey consisted of a series of closed and open-ended questions, and took approximately 20 minutes to complete. The questionnaire was developed with input from community choice counselors and other program staff, Center for State Health Policy staff, and an external reviewer with expertise in long-term care.

The instrument included questions about demographic characteristics, preventive health characteristics, physical ability characteristics, quality of life, health episodes such as emergency room usage and hospitalizations, services, safety, and satisfaction with their current living situation. This chapter reports selected findings from this study.

RESULTS

Current Living Setting

Two of the most important questions that the NJDHSS wanted to know were: where were the people who had been transitioned out of a nursing home living about 2 months later? And, how satisfied were they with that choice?

CSHP found that the majority of clients (80.3%) were living in a home-based setting 8 to 10 weeks after they had been discharged from the nursing home (see Figure 2.2). Within this broad category of "home-based setting," it is interesting to note that the majority were living in their own homes or apartments. Lesser common home-based settings included senior subsidized apartments and someone else's home. Approximately one-fifth of clients (19.7%) were living in other settings (often referred to here as facility-based settings). Nearly one-half these people were living in assisted-living residences (10.4% of the total). A few clients (3.7% of total) were living in nursing homes again.

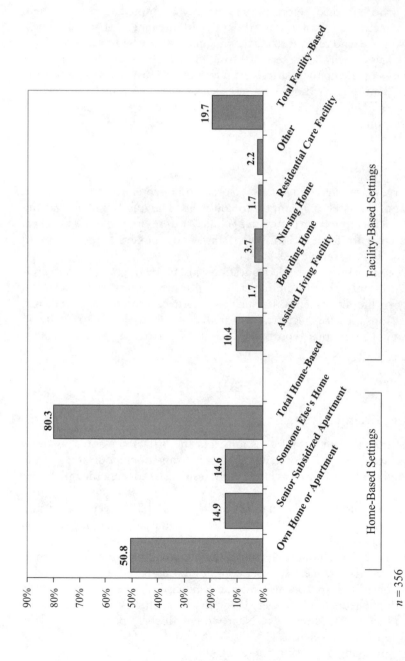

$n = 356$

Figure 2.2   Respondents' Current Living Setting.

It is important to look at the social support of the dischargees living in home-based settings, as the level of support in the community can have an impact on a client's ability to remain in a home-based setting. For instance, clients who have high levels of social support have a larger pool of potential caregivers who can help maintain the client in their home. Of those living in home-based settings, one-third (33.4%) were living alone 2 to 3 months after discharge.

The majority of those living in home-based settings (56.7%) were living with a relative—most often a spouse (19.2%), a daughter (15.3%), or a son (10.1%). Only a few people were living with friends (5.7%), paid caregivers (2.1%), or someone else (1.4%).

The CCC program is based on the belief that people want to have choices and exercise their autonomy—and that no one wishing to stay would be forced to leave a nursing home—but all should be given information and help to live in their preferred setting. Naturally, a question arises—How satisfied were the respondents with their living situation a few months after they moved?

The data indicate that the overwhelming majority of respondents were satisfied with their current living situation. Eighty-nine percent ($n = 310$) of the clients (or their proxies) reported being satisfied with their current living situation.

Only 5% ($n = 19$) voiced dissatisfaction. Because this is such a small number, CSHP did not separate out responses of those who lived in community settings from those who were currently living in nursing homes, boarding homes, or assisted-living facilities. The reasons why these clients or their proxies expressed dissatisfaction included: not liking the setting ($n = 8$), being lonesome ($n = 2$), wanting to be in their own apartment or home ($n = 2$), and feeling unsafe in the neighborhood ($n = 2$).

Activities of Daily Living

Another important question is the extent to which people transferred out of nursing homes are able to perform activities of daily living (ADLs—eating, dressing, bathing, transferring, and toileting) and instrumental activities of daily living (IADLs—using the telephone, mobility, managing medications, managing money, using transportation, housework, meal preparation, laundry, and shopping). This kind of information is helpful in signaling how independent the former nursing home residents are—and may indicate how much they are relying on family and friends.

Although a frail older adult may be able to perform certain activities, they may nonetheless be receiving help with similar or related tasks. For instance, although an older adult may be able to prepare a light meal or snack, their caregiver could prepare his or her main meals. Therefore, respondents were also asked whether they received help with I/ADLs from informal caregivers such as family and friends or from paid caregivers such as home health aides.

In addition, help with certain basic and instrumental activities of daily living may be included in the package of services provided by facility-based living settings such as assisted living facilities. Therefore, CSHP considered the receipt of services only among the home-based population.

ABILITY OR INABILITY TO PERFORM I/ADLS

Because the ability to perform activities of daily living can often influence (as well as be influenced by) one's living situation, the clients' ability to perform ADLs and IADLs was considered separately for home- and facility-based seniors.

On average, the home-based respondents were able to perform 3.7 (SD = 1.8) of the 5 ADLs. One-half were able to perform all 5 ADLs, one-fourth were able to perform up to 4 ADLs, and another one-fourth were able to perform up to 2 ADLs.

With regard to IADLs, on average, the home-based respondents were able to perform 4.3 (SD = 3) of the 9 IADLs. One-half could perform up to 4 IADLs, 15.3% were able to perform all 9 IADLs, whereas 10% could not perform any of the IADLs.

To compare the two groups, on average the facility-based respondents were able to carry out about 3.7 (SD = 1.8) of the ADLs (the same as the home-based group) and 3.4 (SD = 3) of the IADLs (somewhat more dependent than the home-based group). About one-fourth were able to perform up to 2 of the ADLs, one-fourth were able to perform up to 4 ADLs, and one-half were able to perform all 5 ADLs (same as the home-based group). About one-half were only able to perform up to 2 of the IADLs, 14.7% were able to perform all 9 IADLs, whereas 13.3% were not able to perform any of the 9 IADLs.

Activities that presented the greatest difficulty for home-based seniors were transportation (74.4%), shopping (71.9%), laundry (69.7%), housework (67%), preparing meals (58.8%), managing finances (43.0%), bathing (41.5%), and managing medications (40.5%; see Figure 2.3). Facility-based seniors also had difficulty with preparing meals (77.9%), housework (76.1%), laundry (76.1%), transportation (73.1%), managing medications (70.6%), shopping (64.7%), managing finances (64.7%), and bathing (47.1%). Although these activities seemed to present challenges for both home- and facility-based clients, facility-based clients were significantly less able to perform housework ($F = 11.0$, $p < .01$), laundry ($F = 5.2$, $p < .05$), managing finances ($F = 7.8$, $p < .01$), managing

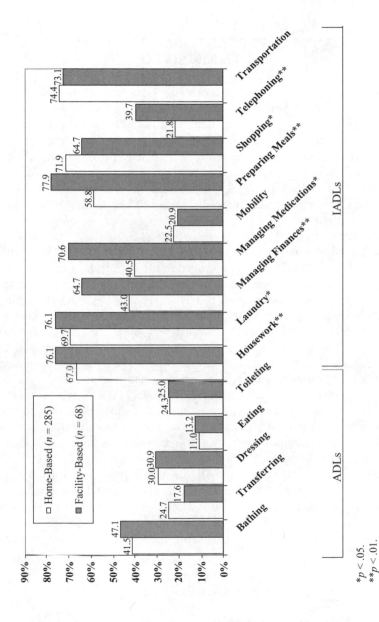

Figure 2.3   Percent of Seniors Unable to Perform ADLs and IADLs (by Type of Activity and Current Living Setting).

*p < .05.
**p < .01.

medications ($F = 17.5$, $p < .01$), preparing meals ($F = 65.7$, $p < .01$), and telephoning ($F = 22.6$, $p < .01$), but were more able to shop ($F = 4.3$, $p < .05$) than the home-based clients.

INFORMAL VERSUS FORMAL CARE FOR I/ADLS RECEIVED

Because home-based seniors can receive services from informal or formal care providers, CSHP assessed the level of care received by type of caregiver as well as type of assistance. Because services are provided as a package for those living in facilities, we report only on the assistance received by the 287 home-based seniors. In general, home-based clients (or their proxies) reported informal assistance with an average of 1.6 (SD = 2) ADLs and 4.9 (SD = 3.3) IADLs. About one-half reported that they did not receive informal care with ADLs, and 1 in 5 reported informal assistance with all five ADLS.

With regard to IADLs, almost one in five (17.8%) home-based seniors did not receive informal help with IADLS, while 18.8% received help with all nine IADLs. Indeed, there was considerable variation in the types of assistance received (see Figure 2.4). Over one-half reported receiving informal assistance with housework (65.1%), laundry (64.9%), managing finances (55%), preparing meals (61.9%), shopping (68.4%), and transportation (68.8%). Additionally, at least one-fourth reported receiving informal assistance with bathing, dressing, transferring in and out of bed, toileting, managing medications, moving around, and using the telephone.

Regarding formal or paid help, home-based respondents reported formal assistance with an average 1.1 (SD = 1.7) ADLs and 1.8 (SD = 2.6) IADLs. Again, it is interesting to note that more than one-half of the clients (62.5%) reported that they did not receive any formal care with ADLs. Not quite one-tenth (9.4%) received assistance with all five activities of daily living.

With regard to IADLs, one-half did not receive any formal help with IADLs. One-fourth received help with one to four IADLs, whereas only 3.7% received formal help with all nine IADLs. Overall, the most frequently used types of formal care included: assistance with bathing (35.5%), housework (30.9%), preparing meals (28.9%), and laundry (28.6%).

MAIN CAREGIVER

One of NJDHSS's major concerns was the impact of nursing home transition on the family caregiver. When asked about their main caregiver, about

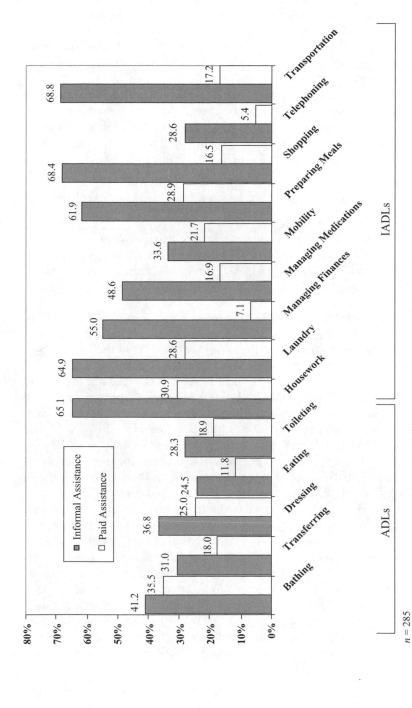

n = 285

Figure 2.4 Percent of Home-Based Seniors Who Receive Informal and Paid Care (by Type of Assistance).

one in four (22.8%) said they cared for themselves (or reported no other caregiver). Most clients (or their proxies) indicated they received informal care from a daughter (16.4%), a spouse (10.5%), or a son (6.6%). Beyond these main caregivers, others less frequently mentioned included friends, grandchildren, multiple family members, and combinations of family and paid caregivers.

Although informal help from family and friends usually suggests unpaid care, that may not always be the case. Therefore, respondents were asked if they paid their informal caregiver. In this sample, almost all informal care was provided without pay, with only 8 seniors paying for help with shopping, and 10 paying for help with transportation.

UNMET NEED WITH I/ADLS

Because so many of those who were helped to leave a nursing home were living in home-based settings, CSHP explored the unmet need for help with ADLs and IADLs. For each ADL and IADL, the researcher asked the client (or proxy) if he or she needed help or needed more help (see Figure 2.5).

The average home-based client needed help (or more help) with approximately one (.98, SD = 1.9) ADL and two (1.8, SD = 3.2) IADLs. It is also interesting to note that three-fourths (74.7%) of the home-based seniors indicated that they did not need additional help.

Although the vast majority of home-based clients did not report any unmet need, a small percentage had significant needs. Approximately one in six people (15.3%) reported needing assistance with all five ADLs. Two-thirds (67.6%) did not indicate needing help (or more help) with any of the nine IADL, whereas 13.2% indicated needing help with all nine IADLs. The most prevalent reported areas of need include transportation (25.2%), bathing (23.8%), housework (23.3%), preparing meals (22.3%), laundry (22.2%), shopping (21.2%), and dressing (20.3%).

Despite the fact that facility-based settings provide case management services, they may not necessarily fill all clients' needs. Therefore, unmet need was also considered for facility-based clients. Almost all of the facility-based seniors reported no unmet needs. Few facility-based clients (or their proxies) reported needing help (or more help), with the average respondent indicating an unmet need in less than one area (0 = .1, SD = 6 for ADLs, 0 = .25, SD = 1.5 for IADLs). Only three clients (or their proxies) reported needing help with ADLs, two reported needing help with one ADL, and one client reported needing help with all five ADLs. Only one client needed assistance with eight IADLS and one needed help with all nine IADLs.

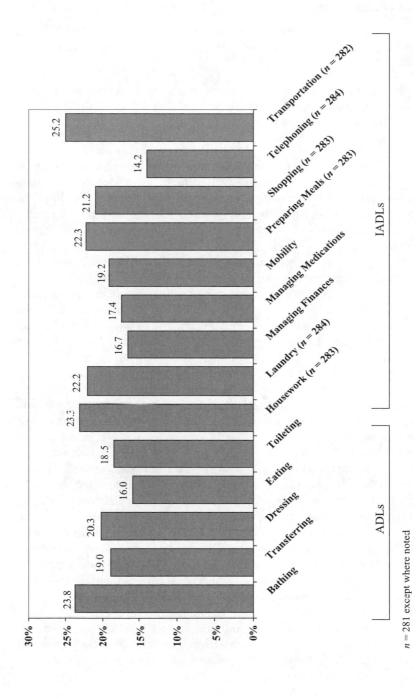

$n = 281$ except where noted

Figure 2.5 Percent of Home-Based Respondents Who Need More Assistance with ADLs and IADLs (by Type of Service).

Total Unmet Needs and Potential Impact of Living Situation

To understand the potential impact of unmet need on the client's living situation, two questions were used to assess the overall adequacy of services:

1. Do you feel that you have the help and services you need to continue living where you are?
2. Do you feel that you have the help and services you need to avoid injury?

In answer to the first question, the majority of clients (or their proxies) was confident that their current level of help was adequate. The data indicate that four-fifths of clients (or their proxies) said that they have the help and services they need to stay where they are. However, a sizable minority ($n = 67$ or 19.1%) expressed some unmet need. Clients or their proxies said that they (or the client) did not have adequate help to stay where they are. Several respondents ($n = 21$) mentioned needing a home health aide or needing 24-hour care ($n = 8$).

Only a few people mentioned needing financial help, respite care, a particular form of therapy, housekeeping, or transportation. When asked why they did not have these services, the two most prevalent responses were lack of finances ($n = 19$) and not knowing whom to contact ($n = 13$).

Another important factor in whether an elderly person is able to remain in the community is whether they are vulnerable to injury. Although DHSS officials expressed the view that it is important to balance risk and independence, they wanted to be sure their program did not put people at undue risk.

When asked if they had the help and services needed to avoid injury, the vast majority 90% ($n = 319$)—said yes. Of the 10% (9.7%, $n = 34$) who felt they did not have the services needed to avoid injury, 14 mentioned needing a home health aide. Other needed services included 24-hour care, a change in their living environment, or a wheelchair. Again, when asked why they did not have the needed services, the most prevalent responses were lack of finances and not knowing whom to contact. Additionally, when the respondents were asked if they (or their proxies) felt safe with their informal caregivers, or paid caregivers, eight individuals reported having concerns.

CSHP attempted to determine the scope of unmet needs of people who had been assisted to leave nursing homes through the following three indicators: needing assistance with ADLs or IADLs, not having the services available to avoid injury, and not having the services needed to remain in one's current setting.

Each of these three dimensions provides specific and often not redundant detail about the area of potential need. For instance, individuals who reported unmet needs for specific forms of assistance did not always consider themselves at risk for leaving their living situations or for injury. Likewise, individuals who felt that unmet needs jeopardized their living situation did not always perceive a threat of injury and did not always mention needing help with specific activities. Overall, one-third of all respondents expressed unmet need in response to at least one of the three approaches (31.1% with the two items and any of the five ADLs, 35.8% with the two items and any of the nine IADLs, 37.8% with the two items and either an ADL or an IADL). More than one in five (20.2%) reported an unmet need that could jeopardize their living situation or expressed concern that they did not have adequate services to avoid injury.

Although limited by the small sample size of facility-based seniors, CSHP also considered whether unmet needs were associated with residential setting. The research team suspected that the important distinctions were between those living in facility-based settings and those living in a home-based setting. Indeed, in the case of facility-based settings there were significant differences for "having the help and services the client needs to continue living where he or she is" ($F = 60.0$, $p < .01$), "having the help and services to avoid injury" ($F = 12.3$, $p < .01$), and reporting at least one unmet I/ADL need ($F = 240.9$, $p < .01$). The people in home-based settings were more likely to report unmet needs on each of the three dimensions.

QUALITY OF LIFE

The goal of the CCC program is to help people choose how they want to live their lives, an important dimension to quality of life. To assess quality of life, the research team asked the former nursing facility residents (or their proxies) three questions:

- Are there activities that you are able to do now that you were unable to do in the nursing home? If so, what activities are you able to do now?
- Are you able to do things that make life enjoyable?
- Are you able to visit with friends and family?

The former nursing home residents were divided evenly concerning whether they could now do things that were not possible in the nursing home: 178 (49.9%) said yes, whereas 179 (50.1%) said no. The activity most reported as gained by having left the nursing home was going out in some fashion such as shopping, visiting, and going for a ride ($n = 50$, 14%). Walking was especially important; of the 50 who mentioned going out in some way, 21 (5.9% of all seniors) specifically referred to being able to go for a walk. Fifteen people (4.2%) had no specific activity in mind, but instead remarked on such benefits as being more independent.

Only 48 (13.4%) of the former nursing home residents mentioned activities they had been able to do in the nursing home that are no longer possible. The activities most commonly mentioned as lost were exercise, physical therapy, or rehabilitation treatment ($n = 15$). Other activities frequently mentioned as being no longer possible in their current living setting were bingo ($n = 5$) and general socializing ($n = 5$).

Beyond activities, the former nursing home residents were asked whether they were able to enjoy their lives. Most people (72.3%) said they are now able to do things that make their lives enjoyable. Of the 31 seniors who mentioned missing activities they had been able to do in the nursing home, 64.6% said their life involved enjoyable activities. The most common activities missing in these seniors' lives, however, seem to be mobility and good health. Among the 93 former residents who said they could not perform activities that make life enjoyable, 26 (7.3% of all respondents) reported problems such as needing assistance to move around or transportation to go out and socialize. Twenty of the former residents (5.6%) said they needed better health to make life enjoyable.

Contact with friends and family is an important aspect of quality of life. The majority of former residents (or their proxies; $n = 301$, 84.3%) said that visiting with family was very important or somewhat important. Visiting friends was important with most ($n = 291$, 81.5%). Although most of the respondents ($n = 251$, 70.3%) said they are able to visit family and friends ($n = 221$, 61.9%), some were less fortunate. Twenty-two former residents (6.2%) said they were not able to visit family because of a physical limitation (including pain and lack of mobility).

Sixteen respondents (4.5%) gave similar reasons for not being able to visit friends. Distance was also a barrier to visiting family ($n = 21$, 5.9%) and friends ($n = 22$, 6%). Not having anyone to visit was also a problem ($n = 16$, 4.5%), with some seniors responding that friends were deceased.

These quality-of-life data indicate that type of housing appears to play little part in overall quality of life. The clients' current residence is not statistically related to enjoyment of life but that measure is related to whom the respondent lives with. Clients living with a relative (including a spouse) were less likely to enjoy life, whereas those living with someone else (other than a family member) were more likely to enjoy life ($X^2 = 10.3$, $p < .05$). People who cared for themselves appear more likely to enjoy life than those being cared for by others ($X^2 = 8.5$, $p < .01$). This relationship holds true regardless of marital status.

OVERALL RESULTS

The CCC program evaluation resulted in several salient research findings:

- Most former nursing home residents are now living in a home-based setting, with the majority of these living with a relative.
- Of those living in a facility setting, most are in assisted-living residences, with only few clients living in nursing homes again.
- Regardless of where they reside, the overwhelming majority of the respondents were satisfied with their current living situation.
- The average home-based senior was able to perform about 4 of the 5 ADLs and 4 of the 9 IADLs. Only 1 in 20 were unable to perform any of the I/ADLs.
- Activities that presented the greatest difficulty were those that were physically and logistically challenging such as bathing, housework, managing finances and medications, and transportation.
- Home-based seniors received most of their assistance from informal caregivers, typically a family member. These caregivers provided help with one-half of the I/ADLs.
- One-half of the clients did not receive any formal care.
- In spite of receiving assistance, the average home-based client indicated needing help (or more help) with about one ADL and two IADLs.
- In contrast, few facility-based clients reported needing help (or more help with I/ADLs).

Although some clients had unmet needs, the majority of clients (or their proxies) were confident that their current level of help was adequate to remain in the community and felt they had the help and services needed to avoid injury. For the minority who didn't have what they needed, most mentioned needing one or more of the following services: a home health aide, 24-hour care, and financial help.

Although the respondents reported these needs, Medicaid does not typically provide all the services that respondents desired such as 24-hour care. Using a three-pronged approach (combining needing assistance with ADLs/IADLs, having the services available to avoid injury, and having the services available to remain in their current setting) provides specific detail about the type of unmet needs these clients may have. And indeed, two-fifths of all respondents expressed unmet need in response to at least one question of the three measures. Using a more conservative approach, namely, considering only those whose unmet needs either jeopardized their living situation or presented a threat of injury, about one in five clients (or their proxies) expressed this level of unmet need.

With respect to quality of life, few former nursing home residents miss the nursing home. Since leaving the nursing home, most seniors report high levels of enjoyment and are able to perform more activities, regardless of the type of current living situation. Additionally, many discharged seniors are able to visit with family and friends, and that increases their quality of life.

Although only minimal information was available on nonrespondents, respondents had significantly shorter lengths of stay in the nursing home than nonrespondents (except for those who were deceased). Therefore, these results should be considered with caution. Nonetheless, the size of this sample of former nursing home residents is sufficient to provide for an appropriate picture of the living situation of those discharged after contact with the CCC program.

CONCLUSIONS

In light of these results, we would like to point out several considerations. Most former nursing home residents are very satisfied when they are helped to leave a nursing home and return to the community. For the most part, they receive the services they need, and have an improved quality of life. Moreover, the community choice counselors (and the program, in general) seem to support and help the nursing home residents' return to the community.

Although the program is successful, there is a group of seniors who report unmet needs that could threaten their continued stay in the community. NJDHSS has developed two new programs, the Caregiver Assistance Program (CAP) and Jersey Assistance Community Caregiving (JACC). These programs provide more flexible community services for both Medicaid (CAP) and non-Medicaid populations (JACC). Although counselors provide information and assistance in setting up community services, we stress the need for clients and their families to be well educated about the type and scope of resources available in the community and whether they are covered under the Medicaid program, even if these services may not be readily available in the community due to high demand. Clients and their families should also be educated to detect changes in the client's situation that may warrant re-examining whether their setting is the most appropriate.

In conclusion, the Community Choice Counseling program seems to be successfully assisting nursing home residents' return to the community with the appropriate set of services. More importantly, seniors are benefiting from an enhanced quality of life by having returned to their community.

REFERENCES

Greiner, P., Snowdon, D., & Greiner, L. (1999). Self-rated function, self-rated health, and postmortem evidence of brain infarcts: Findings from the nun study. *The Journals of Gerontology, 54B*(4), 219–222.

Idler, E., & Benyamini, Y. (1997) Self-rated health and mortality: A review of twenty-seven community studies. *Journal of Health and Social Behavior, 38*(March): 12–37.

Idler, E., Hudson, S., & Leventhal, H. (1999) The meaning of self-ratings of health: A qualitative and quantitative approach. *Research on Aging, 3*, 458–476.

Kane, R. A., Kane, R., & Ladd, R. C. (1998). *The heart of long-term care.* New York: Oxford University Press.

Ladd, R. (1999). *State LTC Profiles Report, 1996. Balancing Long-Term Care.* Minneapolis, MN: Division of Health Services Research and Policy, School of Public Health, University of Minnesota.

Lagnado, L. (2001, February 21). Living and dying: An innovative New Jersey program offers what may be a more humane alternative to nursing homes. *Wall Street Journal*, p. R11.

Nagy, S. Z. (1976). An epidemiology of disability among adults in the United States. *Milbank Memorial Fund Quarterly, 54*, 439–467.

New Jersey Department of Health and Senior Services (NJDHSS). (1991). *Long-term care at the crossroads: Providing options, enhanced quality of life. State health plan proposal.* Trenton, NJ: November 8, 1991.

Reinhard, S., & Scala, M. (2001). *Navigating the long-term care maze: New approaches to information and assistance in three states.* Washington, DC: AARP Public Policy Institute.

Reinhard, S. C., & Fahey, C. J. (2003). Rebalancing long-term care in New Jersey: from institutional toward home and community care [Online]. *Milbank Memorial Fund Quarterly*. Available at www.milbank.org/reports/030314newjersey/030314newjersey#foreword.

CHAPTER THREE

History of and Lessons From the Cash and Counseling Demonstration and Evaluation

Kevin J. Mahoney
Kristin Simone

INTRODUCTION

Currently, in many states, if you are either an elderly individual or a younger person with disability, and if you need assistance through Medicaid to perform activities of daily living like bathing, dressing, toileting, transferring, or eating, you will rarely have much control over who provides services or the scheduling of those services, never mind what services are provided. For years, persons with disabilities have been saying, "If I had more control over my services, my quality of life would improve and I could meet my needs for the same amount of money or less." The Cash and Counseling Demonstration and Evaluation (CCDE), which is described in this chapter, is at its heart, a policy-driven evaluation of this basic belief. CCDE, funded by the Robert Wood Johnson Foundation (RWJF) and the Office of the Assistant Secretary for Planning and Evaluation (ASPE) at the U.S. Department of Health and Human Services, is a test of one of the most unfettered forms of consumer direction—offering consumers a cash allowance to be used toward personal assistance services in lieu of the traditional agency-delivered (controlled) services. Through the CCDE project, consumers are able to choose, hire, and manage their service provider; choose their mix of services; and choose the scheduling of their services. CCDE operates under a research and demonstration waiver granted by the Centers for Medicare and Medicaid Services (CMS).

PROGRAM IMPLEMENTATION PHASES AND CURRENT STATUS

The CCDE has gone through four distinct stages. In this chapter we concentrate on only the first three stages, but near the end we describe the fourth stage.

Stage 1: January 1996 to January 1997: Choosing States and the Evaluator

In January 1996, the University of Maryland Center on Aging (which is coordinating this demonstration on behalf of the RWJF and ASPE) sent out a call for proposals to all states. The volume and quality of the responses were unexpected: 42 states called for additional information; 17 applied, and by the end of 1996, 4 states were chosen—Arkansas, New York, Florida, and New Jersey. Besides having determined which states would participate in the demonstration, the other major accomplishment of the first year was the selection of Mathematica Policy Research, Inc.(MPR) as program evaluator after a national open competition for this critical role. MPR's role was to conduct a quantitative analysis of the impact of the demonstration on the program's major stakeholders, its financial implications, and an evaluation of its implementation strategies.

Stage 2: February 1997 to November 1998: Preparation

Once the players were selected, the planning began in earnest. The "preparation stage" is comprised of five major parts: waiver negotiations, a preference study, policy expert interviews, state infrastructure construction, and protocol development and readiness reviews.

Waiver Negotiations

For the demonstration to proceed, the states needed approval from the CMS for Section 1115 Research and Demonstration Waivers. These waivers freed the states from two Medicaid requirements. The first requirement "waived" through agreement with CMS is that every provider needs to sign an agreement with Medicaid. The second allowed the states to disregard the amount of Medicaid funds a consumer received for personal assistance when determining Medicaid income and resource eligibility. In addition, the individual states had to negotiate approval from SSI and the Food Stamp program to allow members of the treatment group to carry Medicaid personal assistance service (PAS) resources forward from month to month without jeopardizing the consumers' eligibility status for these other vital income supplements.

Preference Study

At the start of the demonstration, the participating states had little notion of how many consumers would be interested in the cash allowance option, which ones, and why. To make an informed decision, they needed to know what type(s) of information consumers and their representatives needed concerning the program and its options. The states also needed to know what types of supportive services consumers desired. To meet these information needs, the RWJF funded a series of focus groups and surveys, which were conducted by the University of Maryland Center on Aging, in each of the four states. The Preference Studies showed that at least half the adults with disabilities and a third of the elderly respondents were interested in learning more about the new option (Simon-Rusinowitz et al., 1998).

Policy Expert Interviews

Faced with the prospect of implementing consumer-directed programs, experts in aging and disability policy helped identify the key issues for consumers, providers, policymakers, and funders. They also explored potential barriers to implementing consumer-directed programs.

The policy experts believed that the key issues for consumers were: consumers need training to manage their care; consumers' preferences for services may differ by age, type of disability, and age of onset; family must be considered in consumer direction; and the risk of abuse and/or neglect by personal care workers may be heightened in the program, without agency monitoring as a safeguard.

Regarding providers, the policy experts identified other issues of concern: agencies fear increased business competition, provider agencies may not accept consumer autonomy, providers are concerned about client competency and agency liability, and independent providers are concerned about employment conditions.

Finally, payers and policymakers had concerns about safety, liability, and accountability surrounding the use of cash in the demonstration (Simon-Rusinowitz, Bochniak, Mahoney, Marks, & Hecht, 2000).

State Infrastructure Construction

Individually, the states had the massive task of designing and operational-izing the outreach, counseling, fiscal intermediary (e.g., bookkeeping and check writing), and quality management components for the demonstra-tion. In addition to the design choices, states had to both procure new providers and contract with them, as well as to make many basic deci-sions including how to cash out the traditional agency-delivered benefits.

States relied on a range of technical assistance activities available from the project's national program office, including expertise in program design, development of the counseling and fiscal intermediary functions, communications, quality management, and information systems design. States also shared information with each other through ongoing meetings and structured technical assistance calls.

Protocol Development and Readiness Reviews

In granting the 1115 Research and Demonstration Waivers, CMS spec-ified 23 terms and conditions relating to monitoring activities, financial reporting, data, and budget neutrality requirements. Each state had to prepare an "Operational Protocol" covering virtually every facet of the demonstration. Once this Protocol was approved, CMS conducted a final "Readiness Review."

Stage 3: December 1998 to June 2003: Implementation/Data Gathering

Within 1 month of having received waiver approval, Arkansas was poised to get underway. New Jersey and Florida took 1 year and $1\frac{1}{2}$ years, respectively, to get up and running. In October 1999, New York was dropped from the demonstration as that state had difficulty recruiting support from Local Social Service Districts and had fallen far behind the evaluation schedule. Table 3.1 summarizes the state of the three remaining states at end of June 2002.

The basic design of the CCDE is the same for each state. Consumers are offered a choice between receiving the traditional agency-delivered PAS services or home-care waiver services listed in their care plans and managing a cash allowance roughly equivalent to the dollar amount of that care plan. Those consumers who volunteer for the demonstration are referred to the evaluator for a baseline interview; they are then randomly assigned either to the treatment group (the cash allowance benefit coupled with a menu of counseling services) or to the control (the traditional agency-delivered services) group. More precisely, Medicaid beneficiaries who are eligible for PAS or waiver services enter the system as they have

Table 3.1 Cash and Counseling at a Glance, June 30, 2002

	Arkansas _Independent Choices_	New Jersey _Personal Preference_	Florida _Consumer-Directed Care_
Implementation date	December 1998	November 1999	May 2000
Populations served	Elderly and adult disabled	Elderly and adult disabled	Elderly, adult disabled, & children w/developmental disabilities
	Medicaid personal care recipients	Medicaid personal care recipients	Medicaid 1915c home- & community-based service waiver clients
Departments involved	Primary: Division of Aging and Adult Services, Department of Human Services. In coordination with: ⇒Division of Medical Services, Department of Human Services	Primary: Division of Disability Services, Department of Human Services. In coordination with: ⇒Division of Medical Assistance & Health Services, Department of Human Services	Primary: Department of Elder Affairs. In coordination with: ⇒Department of Children and Families (Developmental and Adult Services Programs) ⇒Department of Health (Brain and Spinal Cord Injury Program) ⇒Agency for Health Care Administration
Territory covered	Statewide	Statewide	• Central and South Florida—elderly & adult physically disabled • Statewide—children & adults w/developmental disabilities
Enrollment targets*	2,000	2,000	3,000
Final caseload (for evaluation)	2,008 • Adults—556 • Elderly—1,452	1,762 • Adults—821 • Elderly—941	2,820 • Children—1,004 • Adults—1,002 • Elderly—814
Open-enrollment end date	April 30, 2001	June 30, 2002	Children: August 31, 2001 Adults: October 31, 2001 Elderly: June 30, 2002

*Enrollment targets refers to the minimum number of consumers that the evaluator, Mathematica, must interview. Half of the consumers are randomly assigned to the experimental group to receive the cash allowance, whereas the other half are randomly assigned to the control group and remain with traditional services.
Source: www.umd.edu/aging; www.cashandcounseling.org.

done in the past. After receiving a comprehensive assessment, an individualized care plan is developed by caseworkers to meet the client's unmet needs. At this juncture, consumers are given information that will help them to make an informed choice between the "traditional" and the "consumer-directed" options. If he or she opts to be part of the demonstration, (s)he stands a 50–50 chance of being randomly selected to receive the cash allowance. All the people who receive the cash allowance have access to a wide range of counseling services, and these services include assistance with the fiscal tasks associated with being an employer.

The evaluation phase of the demonstration compares outcomes of the treatment and control groups on measures including client satisfaction and quality of care, costs, and differences in the types and amounts of PAS consumers' purchase. The evaluation also examines ways in which the program affects informal caregivers as well as the experiences of paid workers. It includes a study assessing consumers' and their representatives' preferences for traditional or consumer-directed services, a process evaluation, and a counselor feedback questionnaire. In addition, researchers from the University of Maryland, Baltimore County, conducted an in-depth ethnographic study examining 25 triads of consumers/workers/counselors in each state to capture people's experiences with consumer direction.

Several features crosscut each of the demonstration states:

- Consumers must spend their cash allowances only to meet personal assistance needs. Within that framework is considerable flexibility. Each of the three states decided that every consumer would be required to develop a plan for the use of their cash allowance. This was a major decision, as each state understood the need for accountability when using public/Medicaid funds.
- Consumers are allowed to return to the traditional program at any time they wish. If consumers have trouble making consumer direction work but wish to remain in the program, counseling services can be augmented.
- Consumers are assured that they can receive the cash allowance for at least 2 years. (This became an important part of program because planners were concerned whether consumers would make such a major program/plan switch if the cash allowance were offered only for a brief period of time.)
- Consumers who want to be part of the demonstration, but who are not capable of total self-direction, are allowed to have "representatives." What this means in practical terms is that the consumer and his or her representatives share tasks, which include decision making and service management. Representatives are directed to elicit the views/preferences of the consumer and to speak on behalf

of them (as opposed to expressing their own opinions). What this really means is that no one is automatically eliminated from the cash option because of concerns about his or her capacity. Every consumer, it is assumed, is capable of expressing opinions about his or her own care and services.

Even though these three states implemented the same core demonstration, there were important differences in the way they implemented the project. Existing delivery systems affected the way Cash and Counseling was operationalized.

Arkansas contracted with one agency in each region that provided both fiscal and counseling support. New Jersey had a more diversified structure, with outreach consultants, multiple counseling entities, and state program control over changes to the consumer purchasing plans. In Florida, one fiscal intermediary handled the monitoring and payment of the cash plans, but separate counseling approaches were used. For older consumers the program relied on case managers from the area agency network, whereas for consumers with developmental disabilities the local county developmental disability network was used.

Table 3.2 shows how each state divided up the various counseling tasks for the CCDE. It is useful to note how the states differed in the degree to which they integrated counseling and fiscal intermediary (FI) or bookkeeping functions. Arkansas had one agency in each region performing both counseling and FI functions. New Jersey and Florida, believing that there were economies of scale, and that the skills needed for a FI were quite different from the expertise needed to perform counseling duties, selected one FI for the whole state.

In New Jersey and Arkansas, where traditional personal care-provider agencies were their own gatekeepers, the CCDE program felt it was necessary to set up a separate outreach capability to assure that information about CCDE was being delivered in an unbiased manner. In fact, Arkansas and New Jersey chose to establish completely new, parallel delivery systems for Cash and Counseling, whereas Florida attempted to rely on the existing system to the extent possible.

IMPLEMENTATION LESSONS

Coordination of Activities

As a general rule, the greater the number of actors (see Table 3.2), the greater the need for coordination and the longer it took for consumers to start getting the cash allowance. For this reason, the Cash and Counseling states have gradually become convinced that there are real advantages in linking the counseling and FI functions and in using dedicated workers for the consumer-directed option.

Table 3.2 Cash and Counseling: Delivery System Components

	Outreach/ Enrollment	Consumer Training	Cash Plan Development/ Counseling	Cash Plan Approval/ Changes	Fiscal Intermediary (FI)	Monitoring	Reassessment
AR	State		Counseling entity*	Counseling entity*	Counseling entity* (1 per region)	Counseling entity*	Counseling entity*
FL	Counseling entity*	Counseling entity*	Counseling entity*	Counseling entity*	(1) FI	Counseling entity*	Counseling entity*
NJ	For-profit firm specializing in outreach		Counseling entity*	State	(1) FI	Counseling entity* / FI	Medicare RNs

*Counseling entities are organizations that employ professionals who provide cash and counseling supportive services. In some states, the cash and counseling consultants/support brokers were employed by traditional case management agencies; in other cases, organizations specializing in cash and counseling fiscal and support services employed the counselors/consultants.

Outreach and Enrollment

The Cash and Counseling approach is not for everyone. Approximately 15% to 20% of the nonelderly personal-care population in both Arkansas and New Jersey selected this option; in Florida this proportion was closer to 15%. In all three states, approximately 8% to 10% of the eligible elderly individuals chose Cash and Counseling (Phillips, Mahoney, Simon-Rusinowitz, Schore, Barrett, Ditto, Reimers, & Doty, 2003). Although interest in participation in the cash option was lower among the elderly than in the eligible nonelderly individuals, the demonstration has put the myth to rest that elderly people are not interested in consumer direction; 72% of Arkansas' consumer-directed clients are over 65.

In Arkansas, we learned the value of a multifaceted communications plan to stimulate demand. Enrollment can be impacted by outreach (see Figure 3.1). An examination of monthly enrollment figures from Arkansas shows that every time the state made a new outreach effort (e.g., letters to consumers and holiday notes, newsletters, and focus groups with trusted professionals) enrollment numbers sprang up.

In Florida, we learned the advantages of using dedicated outreach workers. Figure 3.2 shows what happened in March 2001 when that state switched to dedicated outreach workers.

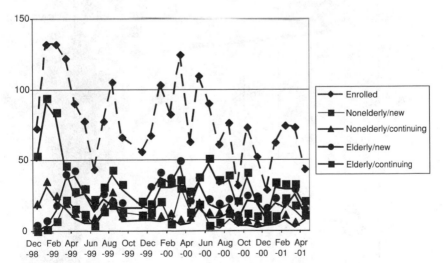

Figure 3.1 Arkansas, Consumer Enrollment in Cash and Counseling: All Groups, April 2001.

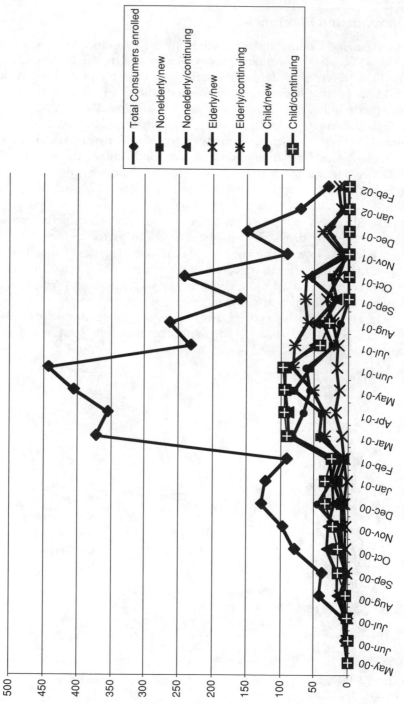

Figure 3.2 Florida, Consumer Enrollment in Cash and Counseling: All Groups, February 2002.

Fiscal Intermediaries

Many of the CCDE's most important early contributions were in procedures for establishing and monitoring FIs. The CCDE has helped develop contracting guides, readiness review criteria, and a template that states can use for monitoring the performance of FIs.

During the first few years of operations, only a handful of consumers have wanted to handle their cash allowances directly. The vast majority of consumers of all ages wanted to use the FI as their "employer agent." In this model, the consumer develops a "cash plan" or individualized budget and instructs the FI on how to spend the cash allowance. With the FI handling the bookkeeping, tax paying, and record-keeping tasks, concerns by policymakers over fraud and abuse have been allayed.

OUTCOMES

MPR (Phillips et al., 2003) released findings from the first 200 to 250 treatment group members completing the 9-month follow-up survey. Already we can see (Table 3.3) that the vast majority of clients in each state would recommend this program to others. Clients (73% to 79%) felt their quality of life was improved a great deal by the Cash and Counseling program, and no one felt they were worse off.

The vast majority of consumers use at least part of their cash allowances to secure personal care attendants and many of these people hire family members and friends (see Table 3.4)

Table 3.3 Satisfaction With Cash and Counseling: Preliminary Results From Interviews With the First 200 Consumers From Each State

| | Percent of Respondents | | |
	Arkansas	New Jersey	Florida
Overall satisfaction			
Would recommend program	93.3	86.1	90.0
How much quality of life was improved			
A great deal	78.7	70.1	73.0
Somewhat	21.3	29.9	27.0
Number of respondents	194	216	219

Source: Foster, L., Brown, R., Carlson, B., Phillips, B., & Schore, J. (2000, 2002a, 2002b) Mathematica Policy Research Inc.'s Nine-Month Cash and Counseling Evaluation Interview.

Table 3.4 Cash and Counseling Demonstration:
Recruiting Methods Resulting in Hires

| | Percent* of Respondents | | |
	Arkansas	New Jersey	Florida
Family member	78.0	63.4	55.3
Friend, neighbor, or church member	15.4	20.4	29.1
Former home care agency worker	1.6	16.1	21.3
By posting/consulting advertisement	0.8	6.5	12.8
Recommended by family/friend	2.4	11.8	19.2
Through an employment agency	0.8	1.1	N/A
Other	0.8	N/A	13.5
Number of respondents	123	93	141

*Percentages total more than 100% as a result of consumers using multiple recruiting methods.
Source: Foster, L., Brown, R., Carlson, B., & Phillips, B., Schore, J. (2000, 2002a, 2002b) Mathematica Policy Research Inc.'s Nine-Month Cash and Counseling Evaluation Interview.

MEDICAID COSTS

Data collected and analyzed by Arkansas (the first state to implement) tell the story. In a comparison of Medicaid beneficiaries who were randomized to receive either the cash option or the traditional Medicaid services, state investigators found:

- Personal-care assistance expenditures were higher for the Cash and Counseling beneficiaries. This may partially be accounted for because the Medicaid beneficiaries in the traditional services group did not receive personal assistance services in 40% of the months during which they were eligible for them, compared to 9% for those in the cash option group.
- Other Medicaid long-term care expenditures were lower among the Cash and Counseling beneficiaries. These other expenditures included those associated with home health services, home and community-based waiver programs, and nursing facilities. Institutional costs were 18% higher for the traditional services group.
- Overall Medicaid costs per recipient per month were virtually identical for the traditional services and the cash option groups.*

---

* Through the first 2 years of operation, the cost per recipient per month for Independent Choices plus the cost per recipient per month for all other Medicaid services was 0.15% less.

WHAT IS NEXT?

Stage 4

The demonstration was so successful that the RWJF and the Department of Health and Human Services, Assistant Secretary for Planning and Evaluation, wanted to continue and expand on the program. In August 2004, the demonstration expanded to 12 additional states. These additional states are Alabama, Illinois, Iowa, Kentucky, Michigan, Minnesota, New Mexico, Pennsylvania, Rhode Island, Vermont, Washington, and West Virginia.

Given the early successes, the Cash and Counseling states are already looking at ways to make this option permanent. We now have sufficient data to measure budget neutrality using trend data based on the experiences of the initial study. The second step might involve broadening Medicaid's definition of "personal care" (so it is no longer limited to human assistance) and amending Medicaid policies governing 1915c waivers to specify how states might incorporate individual budgets into their home and community-based waivers. In the long run, states may find it beneficial to consider operating Cash and Counseling programs through prepaid health plans so they would have the flexibility to advance funds, pay out small amounts of cash, and offer cash allowance alternatives to a wider range of services.

Based on the experiences of Arkansas, Florida, and New Jersey in consumer direction, other states are expanding consumer-directed initiatives and are using individualized budgets to address consumer needs. We hope that these efforts can build on knowledge obtained through Cash and Counseling and make further advances in critical areas such as linking consumers (especially consumers without readily available family members) with workers, developing training for representatives acting on behalf of consumers, and testing quality management approaches (such as the one being developed for the Cash and Counseling states) appropriate for consumer-directed programs.

ACKNOWLEDGMENT

Parts of this chapter were published in early lessons from the Cash and Counseling demonstration and evaluation (2000). *Generations*, 24(3), 41–46.

REFERENCES

Cash and Counseling Web site. www.cashandcounseling.org

Foster, L., Brown, R., Carlson, B., Phillips, B., & Schore, J. (October 2000) Cash and counseling: consumers' early experiences in Arkansas (October 2000). Princeton, NJ: Mathematica Policy Research, Inc.

Foster, L., Brown, R., Carlson, B., Phillips, B., & Schore, J. (April 2002). Cash and counseling: consumers' early experiences in Florida. Part II: Uses of cash and satisfaction at nine months. Interim memo. Princeton, NJ: Mathematica Policy Research, Inc.

Foster, L., Brown, R., Carlson, B., Phillips, B., & Schore, J. (April 2002). Cash and counseling: consumers' early experiences in New Jersey. Part II: Uses of cash and satisfaction at nine months. Interim memo. Princeton, NJ: Mathematica Policy Research, Inc.

Mahoney, K. J., Simone, K., & Simon-Rusinowitz, L. (2000). Early lessons from the cash and counseling demonstration and evaluation. *Generations, 24*(3), 41–46.

Phillips, B., Mahoney, K., Simon-Rusinowitz, L., Schore, J., Barrett, S., Ditto, W., Reimers, T., & Doty, P. (2003). Lessons from the implementation of Cash and Counseling in Arkansas, Florida, and New Jersey. Princeton, NJ: Mathematica Policy Research, Inc.

Simon-Rusinowitz, L., Mahoney, K., Desmond, A., Shoop, D., Squillace, M., & Fay, R. (1998). Determining consumers' preferences for a cash option: Background research to support the Cash and Counseling Demonstration and Evaluation. Synthesis of key telephone survey findings: Arkansas, New York, New Jersey and Florida elders and adults with physical disabilities. Presentation at the 51st Annual Scientific Meeting of the Gerontological Society of America, Philadelphia, PA, November 24.

Simon-Rusinowitz, L., Bochniak, A. M., Mahoney, K. J., Marks, L. N., & Hecht, D. (2000). Implementation issues for consumer-directed programs: A survey of policy experts. *Generations, 24*(3), 34–40.

University of Maryland Center on Aging. Cash and counseling demonstration. (2005). Retrieved June 16, 2005, from www.hhp.umd.edu/AGING/CCDemo/ataglance.html.

CHAPTER FOUR

A Description of Racial/Ethnic Differences Regarding Consumer-Directed Community Long-Term Care

Mark Sciegaj

INTRODUCTION

Historically, federal coverage for disabled individuals moved from cash payments to a vendor payment system in the 1950s as services were increasingly medicalized (Wallack, Sciegaj, & Long, 2002). As a result, most existing public programs that finance personal care services (including Medicaid's optional personal care services benefit and home- and community-based long-term care waiver programs) use agency-based delivery models. Although the degree of consumer involvement varies from program to program, typically under the agency-based model disabled individuals have little control over the management or delivery of their care.

Over the past two decades there has been a growing awareness of the practicality of promoting elder choice and control over community long-term care (CLTC) services (Benjamin & Mattias, 2001; Eustis & Fischer, 1992; Glickman, Stocker, & Caro, 1997; Sabatino & Litvak, 1992; Sciegaj & Capitman, 1994). There have also been numerous strategies proposed for increasing elder participation in the management of their services. For example, some have argued for the adoption of independent living models (DeJong, Batavia, & McKnew, 1992; Simon-Rusinowitz & Hofland, 1993), consumer-directed models (Kapp, 1990; Sabatino, 1990), or cash benefit models (Simon-Rusinowitz, Mahoney, Desmond, Shoop, Squillace, & Fay, 1997) that would allow elders control and choice regarding their services.

Others have suggested reforms within the existing agency-based model such as client-driven quality assurance procedures (Kane & Kane, 1989; Sabatino, 1989) or in-service education of home care providers (Young & Pelaez, 1990) as possible facilitators of elder control and choice.

Although the research literature on elder autonomy, long-term care decision making, and consumer direction has grown in recent years, there remain few studies that have detailed elder preferences for controlling different areas of CLTC services. The few studies available in the literature suggest that elder preferences for control over CLTC services vary. An early study by Cohen (1992) surveyed 57 elders regarding the importance of controlling various details of their care. Cohen's study found the areas of service delivery control considered important to younger adults with disability were not important to frail elders. For example, having control over the hiring, firing, and paying of caregivers was not considered an important element to the elders' sense of independence. What was important to the elders interviewed by Cohen was being able to participate and negotiate their care services schedule.

In addition to supporting the autonomy of elders, a secondary goal of many CLTC programs has been to respect the relationships between the elder and his or her informal caregiver (Dwyer & Coward, 1992; Kemper, Applebaum, & Harrigan, 1987; Sciegaj & Capitman, 1994; Weissert, Cready, & Pawelak, 1988). Although there have been few large studies that have asked elders who they would want to involve in making CLTC decisions, the findings of a study conducted by Blackhall, Murphy, Frank, Michel, and Azen (1995), which explored the role of race/ethnicity in shaping attitudes toward hospital patient autonomy, provide some insight into the relative importance of receiving assistance in CLTC decision making.

Blackhall et al. (1995) conducted interviews with 800 elders evenly divided among African Americans, European Americans, Korean Americans, and Mexican Americans. One topic area covered in these interviews was the following: *Who should make the decision regarding* life-prolonging technology—the patient or the family? Blackhall et al. (1995) reported that Korean American (28%) and Mexican American elders (41%) were less likely to believe that the patient should make the decision than African American (60%) and European American elders (65%). According to Blackhall et al., this finding suggests that Korean Americans and Mexican Americans favor a more family-centered model of medical decision making rather than the more traditional patient autonomy model. Blackhall et al. conclude that physicians should ask their patient whether they wish to receive information and make decisions alone or whether they prefer that their family be involved in this process. Such sensitivity to family involvement is also important to the development of consumer-directed CLTC options for elders, to ensure that the correct party is responsible for making medical choices (Capitman & Sciegaj, 1995; Simon-Rusinowitz & Hofland, 1993).

The lack of consideration of the possible role of race/ethnicity in shaping elder preferences regarding consumer direction in CLTC, and of whether elders' have specific preferences for control over CLTC services, is a major limitation of much current research in this area. The successful expansion of consumer-directed options for elders receiving CLTC will require a better understanding of elders' needs and preferences, and of how race/ethnicity defined subgroups among the potential service population differ. To fill this gap the following study surveyed 731 current elder users of CLTC from four racial/ethnic groups: African American ($n = 200$), Chinese American ($n = 200$), Latino ($n = 131$), and White Western-European American ($n = 200$). The study explored racial/ethnic variation in elder preferences regarding who should (1) make their CLTC decisions, (2) manage their services, and (3) supervise their worker. For each of these questions, elders could respond themselves alone, themselves with assistance from family, or themselves with assistance from an agency staff person (e.g., case manager and social worker).

The study also examined elder preferences among three different CLTC management models: (1) Cash and Counseling Model, (2) Negotiated Care Management or Social Health Maintenance Organization (SHMO) Like Model, and (3) the Traditional Case Management Model. The three models were selected because they offer distinctly different levels of consumer direction. Among these models, high, mid, and low levels of consumer direction were represented. After hearing a description of the three types of models, the elders were asked to rank these in terms of which one they liked the best overall. Follow-up questions probed to what extent elders wanted to have control over various areas of their services. The following sections describe the study methods and present descriptive analyses of elder preferences in consumer direction.

METHODS

Sample

Working with three home- and community-based providers in Boston, Massachusetts, a sample of 731 elders who had at least one daily living impairment were recruited to participate in this study. Included in this number were 200 African American, 200 Chinese American, 131 Latino, and 200 White Western-European American elders. These elders were currently receiving services from the Massachusetts Home Care Program, the Massachusetts Home and Community Medicaid Waiver Program, or Medicaid-financed home health aide services. The study excluded persons who were private pay only, or who were postacute Medicare home health recipients. The 731 elders were interviewed between September 1997 and February 1999.

Procedure

The survey was administered through face-to-face interviews. Interviews lasted between 30 and 40 minutes. Master-level social work and public health students were recruited and trained to administer the survey in the Chinese American, African American, and White Western-European American elder populations. Latino elders were recruited to conduct interviews in that population. The decision to use elders with this last group was based on the prior experiences of the agency of using local community elders in outreach activities. Both the Chinese American and Latino interviews were conducted in the elder's native language with the appropriate dialect. To ensure consistency, all interviewers received technical training in conducting interviews. On completion of the interview, participants received $20.

Measures

The survey instrument developed for this study collected descriptive demographic data as well as health and functional status data. Original measures were created to explore elder preferences for consumer direction and for control in the areas of CLTC service delivery management, worker supervision, and assistance in making CLTC service decisions (Table 4.1). Community-based organizations were recruited to translate the survey instrument into the appropriate dialects for their Latino and Chinese American populations. Then individuals not connected to the community-based organization translated the survey back into English. In addition, small groups of elders from each of the four racial/ethnic groups were used to

Table 4.1 Definitions and Reliability for CLTC Control Scale Measures

Measures and Definition	M (SD)	Reliability*
Service control (range 0–3): Sum of 0 = no, and 1 = yes on three items related to wanting complete control regarding service choices, decisions, and scheduling. The higher the score, the greater the desire for service control.	.98 (1.3)	.91
Worker control (range 0–8): Sum of 0 = no, and 1 = yes on eight items related to wanting complete control regarding hiring, training, and paying service workers. The higher the score, the greater the desire for control over the worker.	.32 (.87)	.85
Decision control (range 0–4): Sum of 0 = wanting assistance, and 1 = wanting complete control on four items regarding service and worker decisions. The higher the score, the greater the desire for making service and worker decisions independently.	.42 (1.1)	.83

*Reliability was measured as internal consistency using Cronbach's Alpha.

pilot-test the survey instrument, and to resolve any potential problems with the overall survey approach.

Items Measuring Elder Preferences for CLTC Service Control and Preference for Consumer Direction

Three measures (Table 4.1) were created to gauge the level of control desired by the respondent over their worker, service package, and CLTC service decisions. A four-item scale was created to measure elder desire for control over CLTC decision making (Cronbach's $\alpha = .83$) incorporating questions regarding the recruitment, hiring, termination, and training of their service worker. A three-item scale measuring desire for control over service planning (Cronbach's $\alpha = .91$) was also created. Questions in this scale asked respondents whether they would want complete control in determining the types of services they receive, making decisions related to their services, and setting their service schedule. Finally, an eight-item scale measuring desire for worker supervision was also created (Cronbach's $\alpha = .85$). Questions in this scale asked respondents whether they wanted responsibility for worker recruitment, training, payment, and the paperwork associated with employment of an individual.

Elder preference for consumer direction was defined as the level of control elders desire in the organization, planning and managing their

Table 4.2 Consumer-Directed Care Model Descriptions

Approach	Description
New Approach 1 (Cash and Counseling Model)	In this approach, you will receive a monthly cash payment, along with some information, training, and advice to help you plan and manage your own care services. In this approach you can also get advice and training from a counselor to learn how to locate, hire, train, schedule, and manage your worker. If you choose, you can also learn how to fill out tax forms for the worker and perform other duties of being an employer. Or, you may have an expert fill out tax forms and do the payment part of the job for you.
New Approach 2 (Negotiated Care Management/ SHMO Like Model)	The agency gives you a set budget based on your needs. Together with the agency you decide what services and what schedule you want. The agency then takes the responsibility for finding and purchasing the services with you.
New Approach 3 (Traditional Case Management Model)	After speaking with you, the agency decides what services and schedule you will get. The agency takes responsibility for choosing, finding, and purchasing the services you need.

CLTC. Respondents were read three brief descriptions of *new approaches* to managing the delivery of their services (Table 4.2) and asked to identify the approach they liked the best overall. New Approach 1 described the Cash and Counseling Model, New Approach 2 described the Negotiated Care/SHMO Like Model, and New Approach 3 described the Traditional Case Management Model.

The Cash and Counseling Model represents one of the most unfettered forms of consumer direction—offering consumers a cash allowance in lieu of agency-delivered services. Individuals in this model can use the cash to purchase services to meet their needs from independent providers, including friends and family if so desired. Also available in this model is a counselor who provides the individual information, training, and advice to assist with planning and managing CLTC services. In addition, the consumer has the option of having a fiscal intermediary agent who attends to paying the CLTC worker and performs other duties associated with being an employer.

The Negotiated Care Management or SHMO Like Model gives the consumer a heightened level of control within an agency service delivery framework. The mechanism for consumer direction in this model is an individual budget for services. How the budget is allocated is negotiated between an agency care manager and the consumer. In this model, the care manager becomes a consultant to and resource for the consumer, helping them to make viable caregiving arrangements (Leutz, Capitman, McAdams, & Abrams, 1992). The meaningful choices of consumers are supported in this program not only by allowing them to express service preferences but also by negotiating their levels of service in response to a known benefit limit (Leutz et al.).

The Traditional Case Management Model is the least consumer directed of the three options. While in this model the consumer is consulted regarding the type and timing of their services, the agency representative has final decision-making power over what services and schedule the consumer receives. The agency also takes responsibility for finding, choosing, and purchasing the services for the consumer.

The survey also collected information regarding sociodemographic characteristics, living situation, health/functional status, desire for information regarding CLTC services, and satisfaction with current services because of their possible influence on elder preferences for consumer direction. Table 4.3 and the following briefly describe these measures.

Living Situation

Because the study was interested in the influence of informal supports on elder preferences for consumer direction, a measure of living situation was created. To determine the living situation, respondents were asked whether they lived alone or, if not, with whom (e.g., spouse, other relative, friend). For analytic purposes, living situation was dichotomized (1 = living alone, 0 = living with others).

Health and Functional Status

Self-assessed health status was measured using the global health assessment question and the Health Perception Scale of the SF-36 (Ware, Snow, Kosinski, & Gandek, 1993). The global health assessment question asks the respondent to assess their health from five possible choices ranking from excellent to poor. For analytic purposes, health status was also dichotomized (1 = excellent/very good/good; 0 = fair/poor). Functional status was measured using the SF-36 Physical Functioning Scale, which asks how limited a person is in 10 activities such as running, walking, lifting, carrying, climbing stairs, bathing, and dressing. Depending on an individual's limitations, the scale ranges from 10 (very limited) to 30 (not limited). The psychometric properties of the scales making up the SF-36 are well documented, and the Cronbach's alpha ($\alpha = .87$) found in this study is consistent with the reported literature (McHorney, Ware,

Table 4.3 Definitions and Reliability for Other New Scale Measures

Measures and Definition	Mean (SD)	Reliability*
General locus of control		
(Range 5–25): Sum of 1 = strongly agree, 2 = agree, 3 = neither agree nor disagree, 4 = disagree, 5 = strongly disagree on five items related to general control in one's life. The higher the score, the greater the sense of being in control.	15.7 (3.8)	.69
Desire for information		
(Range 0–4): Sum of 0 = no, and 1 = yes on four items related to desire to receive information on service providers, types of services available, workers, and the experiences of others. The higher the score, the greater the desire for information.	1.4 (1.4)	.84
General service satisfaction		
(Range 7–35): Sum of 1 = strongly agree, 2 = agree, 3 = neither agree nor disagree, 4 = disagree, 5 = strongly disagree on seven items related to amount, type, and scheduling of services, ability to change service package, current involvement in service selection, decisions regarding service amount, and scheduling decisions.	15.3 (5)	.82

*Reliability was measured as internal consistency using Cronbach's Alpha.

& Raczek, 1993; McHorney, Ware, Rogers, Raczek, & Lu, 1992; Ware, Kosinski, Baylis, McHorney, Rogers & Raczek, 1995).

Service Satisfaction

Two measures of service satisfaction were originally created. First, a four-item scale was developed to measure the respondent's overall satisfaction with current CLTC services (Cronbach's $\alpha = .82$). Items included questions regarding satisfaction with amount, type, and timing of services and the respondent's ability to make changes to service arrangements. Second, a three-item scale was created to measure elder satisfaction with their control over current CLTC services (Cronbach's $\alpha = .82$). Items included questions regarding satisfaction with involvement in deciding the amount, type, and timing of services. Because these two individual scales were highly correlated (Pearson's correlation = .68, $p = .000$), the scales were combined to make a measure of service satisfaction (Cronbach's $\alpha = .84$).

Desire for Information

Because it is generally accepted that elder consumers need adequate information to make meaningful CLTC decisions (Kane, Degenholtz, & Kane, 1999), a four-item desire for information measure was developed (Cronbach's $\alpha = .84$). Items included questions regarding whether the respondent would like to receive information regarding types of services available to them, information concerning service agencies and workers, and the experiences of others with either these services or providers.

Locus of Control

A measure was created to gauge the level of control respondents felt they had over their lives. This measure was created because the study assumed that elder preferences are shaped in part by the particulars of the individual's situations including (1) how they perceive their care needs, (2) their understanding of the range of choices available to them to satisfy these needs, (3) what makes for a meaningful choice among the available options, and (4) how their decisions are considered and respected (or not) by others. To measure the respondent's sense of general control in their lives, a five-item scale was created that included three items from a Mastery Scale developed by Pearlin, Lieberman, Menaghan, and Mullan (1981) as well as two additional new questions (Cronbach's $\alpha = .69$).

To determine the relationship between the new measures created for the study, a correlation matrix was created (Table 4.4). As reported in Table 4.4, Desire for Service Control has a strong correlation with Desire for Information (Pearson's correlation $= .42$). Also, Desire for Service Control and Desire for Decision Control have strong relationships with Desire for Worker Control (Pearson's correlation $= .48$; Pearson's correlation $= .42$, respectively). However, none of the correlation scores between these measures indicate they are measuring the same construct.

RESULTS

For the descriptive analysis, one-way analysis of variance (ANOVAs) and chi-square tests were performed to compare differences among the four groups. In addition, Duncan's post-hoc tests were computed to examine statistical differences between the racial and ethnic groups. Significant differences were found between the groups with respect to demographic

Table 4.4 Correlation Between New Consumer-Directed Measures

	Locus of Control	Desire for Service Control	Desire for Worker Control	Desire for Decision Control	Desire for Information	General Service Satisfaction
Locus of control	1.00					
Desire for service control	−.018	1.00				
Desire for worker control	.104*	.489**	1.00			
Desire for decision control	.191**	.337**	.427**	1.00		
Desire for information	−.058	.426**	.224**	.102*	1.00	
General service satisfaction	.002	.159**	.011	.053	.118*	1.00

*$p < .01$.
**$p < .001$.

characteristics (e.g., age, marital status, and living situation), health and functional status, general locus of control, desire for CLTC service information, desire for CLTC control (e.g., control over services, worker, and decisions), and preferences for consumer direction (Table 4.5, Figure 4.1).

Demographic Characteristics

On average, the Chinese American elders in this study were the oldest ($M = 80$), reporting the highest percentage of being married (37%) and living alone (60%). The Latino elders reported being the youngest ($M = 75$), having the most functional limitations ($M = 13$) and the fewest number (4%) reporting to be in "good health." There were no significant differences between the groups with respect to gender. The majority of respondents within groups were female, and for the total sample, 73% were female.

Sense of Control, Satisfaction, and Desire for Information

There were significant differences between the groups with regard to locus of control with the Chinese American elders reporting the greatest sense of control in life ($M = 17$) and the Latino elders the least ($M = 13$). Perhaps

Table 4.5 Sociodemographic and Attitude Characteristics of Respondents

Characteristic	African American N = 200 M(SD) or %	Chinese American N = 200 M (SD) or %	Latino N = 131 M (SD) or %	White Western-European American N = 200 M (SD) or %	Total sample N = 731 M (SD) or %
Demographics					
Age*	77.4 (7.7)	80 (7.7)	74.7 (7.6)	77.1 (7.4)	77.6 (7.6)
Female	73.6	72.7	68.7	70.6	72.7
Married**	5	37	21	14	19
Living alone**	32.1	59.6	16	29.9	72.6
Functional status					
Good health**	44.9	16.9	3.7	34.6	20
Functional limitations**	16.3 (4.72)	15.7 (4.67)	13.5 (3.82)	17.2 (4.12)	16.1 (4.60)
Satisfaction/control					
General Locus of Control score**	16.7 (3.84)	17.3 (3.48)	13.1 (2.76)	15.3 (3.74)	15.7 (3.8)
General Service Satisfaction score	15.5 (5.5)	15.3 (3.2)	15.4 (5.9)	15.4 (4.8)	15.2 (4.9)
Desire for Information Score*	1.7 (1.42)	.05 (1.15)	2.7 (1.21)	1.2 (1.23)	1.2 (1.46)
Desire for CLTC control					
Desire for service Control score**	1.0 (1.23)	.26 (.84)	2.4 (1.28)	.73 (1.13)	.98 (1.34)
Desire for worker Control score**	.92 (1.07)	.30 (.86)	.73 (.74)	.40 (.68)	.32 (.87)
Desire for Decision Control Score*	.72 (1.44)	.23 (.87)	.29 (.93)	.39 (.94)	.42 (1.10)
Preferences for consumer direction					
New Approach 1	9	3	2	8	6
New Approach 2*	18	47	10	16	24
New Approach 3*	73	50	88	76	70

Note: Chi-square tests for categorical variables; ANOVA for continuous variables with Duncan's post-hoc tests.
* p < .01.
** p < .001.

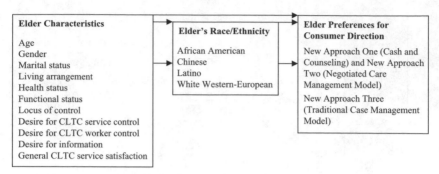

Figure 4.1 Analytic Model.

because of this, it was not surprising to find that the Latino elders expressed the strongest desire for information about services and providers ($M = 3$). There were no significant differences between the groups regarding satisfaction with current services. The percentage of elders in this study who were either satisfied or very satisfied with their care or their involvement with decisions surrounding their care was 85%.

Desire for CLTC Control and Consumer Direction

There were significant group differences for the three CLTC measures of control. Latino elders expressed the strongest desire for control over their services ($M = 2.4$). African American elders expressed the strongest desire for control over their workers ($M = .92$) and for making decisions regarding their services without assistance from family or professional agency staff ($M = .72$). Table 4.5 also reports elder preferences for the different *new approach* models described earlier. With the exception of the Chinese American elders, the overwhelming majority of African Americans ($n = 146$; 73%), Latinos ($n = 116$; 88%) and White Western-European Americans ($n = 152$; 76%) preferred the Case Management Model (New Approach 3). Only half the Chinese elders ($n = 100$; 50%) preferred this model. However, across elders in this study, a significant percentage ($n = 217$; 30%) preferred a more consumer-directed approach (either Cash and Counseling or the Negotiated Care Model). As reported in detail elsewhere (Sciegaj, Capitman, & Kyriacou, 2004), even after controlling for other significant variables, there remained significant racial/ethnic differences for CLTC control and consumer direction.

To further explore the desire, among groups of elders, for control in the aforementioned three CLTC service areas and preferences for consumer direction, elders were asked to indicate which activities they wanted *complete control over*. As reported in Table 4.6, there were significant

Table 4.6   Racial/Ethnic Preferences for Complete Control Over Service Areas

	African American (n = 200) %	White (n = 200) %	Chinese (n = 200) %	Latino (n = 131) %
Service decisions	22	14	6	3
Service schedule	17	13	5	4
Recruiting worker	8	2	4	3
Hiring/firing worker	10	5	4	4
Training worker	10	3	3	5
Paying worker	7	4	2	12

racial/ethnic differences with respect to wanting complete control over CLTC decisions, services, and worker-related issues. With regard to CLTC decisions, 22% of the African American elders and 14% White Western-European American elders wanted to make these decisions independently of either family or professional staff; whereas only 6% of Chinese American and 3% of Latino elders wanted this type of independence. Likewise 20% of African American and 15% of White Western-European American elders wanted complete control over selecting the type of services they received, whereas smaller percentages of Chinese American (5%) and Latino (5%) elders wanted complete control over service selection. Finally, 17% of African Americans and 13% of White Western-European American elders wanted complete control over the scheduling of their services. Again, much smaller percentages of Chinese American (5%) and Latino (4%) elders wanted this level of control.

Much smaller percentages of elders wanted complete control over the CLTC service worker (Table 4.6). Eight percent of African Americans wanted complete control over recruiting the worker. Only 4% of Chinese American, 3% of Latino, and 2% of the White Western-European American elders wanted to have complete control in this area. Ten percent of African American elders wanted complete control over hiring and firing the worker and 10% wanted complete control over worker training. When it came to having complete control over paying the worker, only 7% of the African American elders wanted this type of control, but 12% of Latino elders (more than double the percentage for any other area of control) indicated they would want complete control.

Table 4.7 reports on the same items but instead of racial/ethnic groups it considers elders' desire for complete control between stated preferences for consumer direction. Not surprisingly, elders who preferred the Cash and Counseling Model reported the highest percentages of wanting complete control in the areas of decisions, services, and worker. However, what is interesting to note are the significant percentages of elders who

Table 4.7 Elder Desire for Complete Control by Stated Preferences for Consumer Direction

	Cash and Counseling Model (n = 42)%	SHMO Model (n = 169)%	Traditional Case Management Model (n = 520)%
Service selection	66.0	27.8	34.2
Service decisions	69.0	27.2	33.8
Service schedule	59.7	19.0	31.9
Recruiting worker	31.0	10.7	9.0
Hiring/firing worker	28.6	10.1	6.3
Training worker	31.0	8.3	5.0
Paying worker	26.2	6.5	2.3

preferred the traditional case management model but who also expressed a desire to have complete control over CLTC decisions (34%), service selection (34%), and service scheduling (32%). This finding seems to suggest that although elders may prefer an agency model (and the security it affords) they also want to be in control in aspects of their care management. In other words, consumer direction should not be seen as an all or nothing prospect.

Also of interest are the high percentages of elders (not in table) who preferred the Cash and Counseling Model who wanted either family or agency personnel participation in service scheduling (40%), selection (34%), and service decisions (30%). When considering worker-related issues, approximately 70% of elders who preferred Cash and Counseling also wanted assistance in recruiting (69%), hiring/firing (71%), training (69%), and payroll-related activities (74%). These high percentages also seem to suggest that even when an elder states a preference for a model designed to be more (or less) consumer directed, this means they desire either total control or total passivity regarding their involvement with care management and or service delivery.

DISCUSSION

Although the interpretation of the findings is constrained by the descriptive nature of analyses and some important study limitations, to be discussed, the findings presented here suggest two main conclusions. First, elder preferences for CLTC service control and consumer direction span a continuum. Second, differences between and within racial/ethnic groups do exist. Before discussing these conclusions, the following study limitations need to be noted. These limitations include potential bias in the recruited sample and in the presentation of the alternative consumer direction models.

First, the respondents were recruited from three community-based agencies noted for their cultural competency. Elders receiving services from these organizations typically have case managers and direct care workers who can communicate in their native language or are of the same race/ethnicity. It was not surprising, therefore, that the percentage of elders in this study who were either satisfied or very satisfied with their care or their involvement with decisions surrounding their care was 85%. Furthermore, there was no significant difference in the percentage of elder satisfaction between racial/ethnic groups. This satisfaction with their current care (a traditional case management approach) might explain why 71% of elders in this study selected the Traditional Case Management Model (New Approach 3).

A second study limitation is that the elders were presented with only hypothetical models regarding consumer direction in CLTC. If, however, these elders were selected to participate in the Cash and Counseling Demonstration, they would have received more information than provided in this survey. They also would have had an opportunity to discuss their options with trained case managers. It is not clear whether elder preferences for the different consumer-directed models used in this study would be the same if the elder was indeed required to make a decision regarding consumer direction in CLTC, or if they had more time to reflect on the differences in each model. Even with these limitations, the findings of this study do provide some insight for individuals interested in the development of consumer-directed care models for elders.

Consumer Direction is a Continuum

At its essence, consumer direction attempts to give individuals greater control over the management and delivery of their CLTC services. When examining the effects of control, research on elders often overlooks the possibility that individuals may wish to exercise more control in some domains of their life than in others (Bisconti & Bergeman, 1999). For example, Diwan, Berger, and Manns (1997) report CLTC recipients may reject one service because they want a family member to do it, but that same client may want to accept control over other services. Certainly, the findings of this study suggest that elders who desire more control in one area of their CLTC service delivery *may not* desire more control over all areas. The percentages reported earlier are certainly in keeping with other published observations suggesting elders' preferences for the amount of control they want in service planning and management are complicated and not a simple *all-or-nothing* proposition (Capitman & Sciegaj, 1995; Cohen, 1992; Eustis & Fischer, 1992; Sciegaj et al., 2004).

The Importance of Considering Racial/Ethnic Heterogeneity

The study findings reveal that although racial/ethnic group membership might influence the elder's preference for CLTC service control or consumer direction, heterogeneity also exists within the groups. The findings reported here seem to confirm the importance of looking beyond global racial/ethnic variables and support recent publications regarding the importance of examining the interaction of race/ethnicity with other life situational or attitudinal factors (Angel & Angel, 1997; Burlingame, 1999; Mui, Choi, & Monk, 1998; Valle, 1998). As Angel and Angel articulate, race/ethnicity may give elders a structure through which to view the world; however, it does not necessarily dictate behavior. Three recent reviews on this topic conclude that race/ethnicity competes with other factors in determining individual preferences for how elders live their lives, address illness and care, and what kind of help they desire (Burlingame 1999; Mui et al., 1998; Valle, 1998). These authors point out that a truly sophisticated view of race/ethnicity and its impact on an elders' needs and preferences requires an understanding of its interaction with other factors that have a significant impact on their life and social context.

Therefore, the results of the study indicate that it is important to provide elder consumers with a range of options that might allow for greater control in a variety of *areas* of CLTC service delivery. This knowledge can then lead to the development of different approaches and care planning strategies. Such an informed empathy among care managers and elder CLTC consumers can close the gap between the elders' perceptions and preferences and their professional perceptions and judgments.

The findings of this study can be very useful to current discussions regarding the development of consumer-directed care models for elders in a number of critical areas.

For example, information on the contextual implications of race/ethnicity on elder preferences can prepare case managers to assume differences in worldviews between themselves and the older consumer. The study findings suggest that although a greater appreciation of the role of race/ethnicity is imperative, it only explains part of the picture of how elders live their lives, address illness and care, and what kind of help they desire. Further study is needed to develop a more sophisticated understanding of race/ethnicity and its impact on an elder's needs and preferences.

REFERENCES

Angel, R., & Angel, J. (1997). *Who will take care of us? Aging and long-term care in multicultural America.* New York: New York University Press.

Bisconti, T. L., & Bergeman, C. S. (1999). Perceived social control as a mediator of the relationships among social support, psychological well-being, and perceived health. *The Gerontologist, 39*(1), 94–103.

Benjamin, A. E., & Matthias, R. E. (2001). Age, consumer direction, and outcomes of supportive services at home. *The Gerontologist 41*(5), 632–642.

Blackhall, L., Murphy, S., Frank, G., Michel, V., & Azen, S. (1995). Ethnicity and attitudes towards patient autonomy. *Journal of the American Medical Association. 274*(10), 820–829.

Burlingame, V. S. (1999). *Ethnogerocounseling: Counseling ethnic elders and their families.* New York: Springer Publishing Company.

Capitman, J., & Sciegaj, M. (1995). A contextual approach for understanding individual autonomy in managed community longterm care. *The Gerontologist, 35*(4), 533–540.

Cohen, E. (1986). *Enhancing personal autonomy of disabled elderly.* Narberth, PA: Community Services Systems, Inc.

Cohen, E. (1992). What is independence? *Generations.* Winter, 49–52.

DeJong, G., Batavia, A., & McKnew, L. B. (1992). The independent living model of personal assistance in national long-term care policy. *Generations.* Winter, 89–95.

Diwan, S., Berger, C., & Manns, E. K. (1997). Composition of the home care service package: Predictors of type, volume, and mix of services provided to poor and frail older people. *The Gerontologist, 37*(2), 169–181.

Dwyer, J. W., & Coward, R. T. (Eds.). (1992). Gender, families, and eldercare. Newbury Park, CA: Sage Publications, Inc.

Doty, P., Kasper, L., & Litvak, S. (1996). Consumer-directed models of personal care: Lessons from Medicaid. *Milbank Quarterly, 74*(3), 377–409.

Eustis, N. N., & Fischer, L. R. (1992). Common needs, different solutions? Younger and older homecare clients. *Generations, 16*(1), 17.

Glickman, L. L., Stocker, K. B., & Caro, F. G. (1997). Self-direction in home care for older people: A consumer's perspective. *Home Health Services Quarterly, 16*(1/2), 41–54.

Kane, R. A., Degenholtz, H. B., & Kane, R. L. (1999). Adding values: An experiment in systematic attention to values and preferences of community long-term care clients. *Journals of Gerontology: Social Sciences, 54B*(2), S109–S119.

Kane, R., & Kane, R. (1989). Reflections on quality control. *Generations,* Winter, 63–69.

Kapp, M. (1990) Home care client-centered systems: Consumer choice vs. protection, *Generations,* 14 (Suppl.): Winter, 33–35.

Kemper, P., Applebaum, R., & Harrigan, M. (1987). Community care and demonstrations: What have we learned? *Health Care Financing Review, 8*(4): 87–100.

Leutz, W., Capitman, J. A., MacAdam, M., & Abrahams, R. (1992). *Care for frail elders: Developing community solutions*. Westport, CT: Auburn House.

McHorney, C. A., Ware, J. E., & Raczek, A. (1993). The MOS 36-Item Short Form Health Survey (SF36): II. Psychometric and clinical tests of validity in measuring physical and mental health constructs. *Medical Care, 31*(3), 247–263.

McHorney, C. A., Ware, J. E., Rogers, W. H., Raczek, A. E., & Lu, J. F. R. (1992). The validity and relative precision of MOS short- and long-form health status scales and Dartmouth COOP charts: Results from the Medical Outcomes Study. *Medical Care, 30*(Suppl. 5), MS253–MS265.

Morris, R., Caro, F. G., & Hansen, J. E. (1998). *Personal assistance: The future of home care*. Baltimore, MD: Johns Hopkins University Press.

Mui, A. C., Choi, N. G., & Monk, A. (1998). *Long-term care and ethnicity*. Westport, CT: Auburn House.

Pearlin, L., Lieberman, M., Menaghan, E., & Mullan, J. (1981). The stress process. *Journal of Health and Social Behavior, 22*, 337–356.

Sabatino C. (1989). Home care quality. *Generations*, Winter, 12–16.

Sabatino, C. (1990) *Lessons for enhancing consumer-directed approaches in home care*. Washington D.C.: The Commission on Legal Problems for the Elderly.

Sabatino, C. P., & Litvak, S. (1992). Consumer-directed homecare: What makes it possible? *Generations, 14*(3), 55–58.

Sciegaj, M., & Capitman, J. (1994). *Respecting individual autonomy in managed community long-term care systems: Report to the Office of Technology Assessment, United States Congress*. Waltham, MA: Institute for Health Policy, Heller Graduate School, Brandeis University.

Sciegaj, M., Capitman, J. A., & Kyriacou, C. K. (2004). Consumer-directed community care: Race/ethnicity and individual differences in preferences for control. *The Gerontologist, 44*(4), 489–499.

Simon-Rusinowitz, L., & Hofland, B. (1993). Adopting a disability approach to home care service for older adults. *The Gerontologist, 3*(2), 159–167.

Simon-Rusinowitz, L., & Mahoney, K. J. (2001). *Preferences for consumer-directed services among different consumer groups: Cash and counseling demonstration and evaluation early findings*. Paper presented at Independent Choices: A National Symposium on Consumer-Direction and Self-Determination for the Elderly and Persons with Disabilities, June 10–12.

Simon-Rusinowitz, L., Mahoney, K. J., Desmond, S. M., Shoop, D. M., Squillace, M. R., & Fay, R. A. (1997). Determining consumer preferences for a cash option: Arkansas survey results. *Health Care Financing Review, 19*(2), 73–96.

Valle, R. (1998). *Caregiving across cultures*. Washington, DC: Taylor and Francis.

Wallack, S., Sciegaj, M., & Long, L. (2002) Short and intermediate term trends affecting Medicaid policy for persons with disability, chronic illness, and special needs. *The Journal of Disability Policy Studies, 12*(4), 236–242.

Ware, J. E., Kosinski, M., Bayliss, M. S., McHorney, C. A., Rogers, W. H., & Raczek, A. (1995). Comparison of methods for scoring and statistical analysis of SF26 health profiles and summary measures: summary of results from the Medical Outcomes Study. *Medical Care*, *33*(Suppl. 4), AS264–AS279.

Ware, J. E., Snow, K. K., Kosinski, M., & Gandek, B. (1993). *SF-36 Health survey manual and interpretation guide*. Boston, MA: New England Medical Center, The Health Institute.

Weissert, W.G., Cready, C. M. & Pawelak, J. E. (1988). The past and future home- and community-based long-term care. *Milbank Memorial Fund Quarterly*, 66(2): 309–88.

Young, P., & Pelaez, M., (1990). Ethical education of home-care providers. *Generations*. Supplement, 1990.

CHAPTER FIVE

Case Managers' Perspectives on Consumer Direction

Suzanne R. Kunkel
Ian M. Nelson

Over the past decade, the growth of consumer direction as a model of service delivery for older people has been dramatic. Three-fourths of the 40 states responding to a survey offer consumer-directed home and community-based services; 20 states offer two or more consumer-directed options within their home-care system for older adults (Infeld, 2004). As a growing trend in long-term services for older people, consumer direction (CD) has implications for consumers, their families, workers, clinical professionals, and service agencies. One of the greatest challenges, and greatest hopes, for consumer direction as a service option is to integrate this approach into existing case-managed programs. In such programs, case managers are crucial to the success of CD. For this reason, the perspective of case managers on the realities of implementing CD is invaluable. Case managers provide the initial training and the tools to support the consumers who enroll in the program, and they see firsthand which approaches work and which do not. The role of case managers becomes more complex and multifaceted in the case of self-directed clients, continuing a trend in the evolution of case management as a profession that must be flexible, dynamic, clinically sound, and responsive to consumers.

The expansion of CD into traditional case management structures raises the possibility of either "common ground or contested terrain" between the philosophies and professional practice standards of case management and the goals of consumer self-direction (Kunkel,

Duffy-Durham, & Scala, 2000). A recently completed CD demonstration project provides insights into strategies for, and challenges of, blending self-direction and case management. The Consumer-Directed Care (CDC) option was opened to participants receiving services from a tax-levy-funded home-care program in southern Ohio. In CDC, consumers hire and manage their own workers and direct their own services. For consumers, case managers are the first point of contact about the new option; they provide training to consumers who choose to self-direct; and they continue to provide care planning, assessment, and ongoing support for their consumer-directed clients. This paper reviews the intersection of consumer direction and case management and presents findings from the CDC demonstration to shed light on this issue. Specifically, we present data from a survey of a cross-section of case managers about their attitudes about consumer direction. This survey was conducted a few months before the CDC option was implemented. We also present findings from case manager focus groups conducted 1 year after consumers began to enroll in self-direction.

CASE MANAGEMENT AND CONSUMER DIRECTION: THE TWAIN SHALL MEET

CD arose during the 1970s as part of the independent living movement for younger adults with disabilities (Scala & Mayberry, 1997). In the late 1980s, CD began to move into the area of long-term care services for older adults, although adoption of this concept was initially slow. This slow implementation may have been due, in part, to a long-term care system that emphasizes safety, protection, and the provision of professional supervision of services for older consumers (Schneider, Mahoney, & Simon-Rusinowitz, 2001).

Despite a later start, CD is taking root in home care for older adults; some of the recent growth is occurring in programs that include traditional case management services. In a recent study of 40 states, 68% of the consumer-directed programs offered traditional case management services (Infeld, 2004). The basic philosophy of CD is that people with disabilities (including older people) have the capacity *and* the right to assess their own needs; determine how, when, where, and by whom those needs should be met; and continuously assess and improve the quality of the services they are receiving.

This philosophy contrasts with views of traditional case management as "an intervention using a human service professional to arrange and monitor an optimum package of long-term care services" (Applebaum

& Austin, 1990). Traditional case management emerged as a method to assist individuals with the coordination of needed long-term care services. Due to a fragmented and complex system, older adults were faced with serious obstacles as they tried to access services (Applebaum & Austin). Many of the services they needed required several different providers, and often multiple funding sources (such as Medicaid waivers, Older Americans Act, and Medicare). Case managers have the clinical skills, professional training, experience with the service system, and a commitment to beneficence—doing good for others; all of these are useful skills and characteristics to provide the assistance needed by older people in navigating the complex system. However, this combination of attributes can tip the scales in favor of the primacy of professional expertise, client safety, and minimal risk; in contrast, consumer direction places greater emphasis on client independence and autonomy (Kunkel, Duffy-Durham, & Scala, 2000).

Given the philosophy of CD, it is clear that the case manager role is certainly affected. Even though case managers espouse a sincere respect for client voice, the balance of responsibilities and authority does change in consumer direction. In the national Cash and Counseling demonstration, the use of titles such as counselor, consultant, and support broker speaks to this shift in emphasis. These titles reflect a fundamental change in the roles of consumers and professionals. Even though some consultants/counselors in the Cash and Counseling program are trained as case managers, when they are working with self-directed clients, they fill a different function—emphasizing coaching, training, and supporting the client, rather than intervening on their behalf.

Early research on CD revealed concerns from case managers regarding their changing role. Case managers within one independent living program expressed ambivalence about whether increased risks to consumers would be offset by gains in autonomy (Micco, Hamilton, Martin, & McEwan, 1995). Many case management concerns stem from the inability to let go of a sense of responsibility for clients. As noted previously, case managers traditionally intervene on behalf of their clients; consumers give input, but the traditional assumption is that professional training and experience gives the case manager more expertise in care planning and service management than the client. The beneficence that is an underlying value of case management can manifest as maternalism toward clients. CD calls that value into question. Although case managers want to encourage consumer autonomy, they worried about who would monitor client services to prevent fraud, misuse of funds, or substandard quality of care (Scala, Mayberry, & Kunkel, 1996).

CASE MANAGEMENT AND CONSUMER DIRECTION: THE TWAIN DO MEET

The Council on Aging of Southwestern Ohio (CoA) began the CDC pilot project in 2001, offering the option to clients in the Elderly Services Program (ESP) in two counties. ESP is a tax-levy-funded home-care program, serving approximately 3,900 clients. The target population for the ESP program is individuals with significant need for assistance who do not meet the Medicaid-waiver income and need eligibility requirements. Case managers coordinate all home-care services for the client and are required to see the client at least twice a year. The CDC option was open to all ESP clients, with an enrollment limit of 150 clients for the two counties.

Nine ESP case managers volunteered to participate in the design and early implementation of the new option. These case managers maintained their traditional client caseload as well as their new CDC clients. During the initial discussions about CDC, these care managers expressed some concerns (sometimes on behalf of their colleagues who were not participating in the design phase). Mirroring the tensions described by case managers in previous research on consumer direction, these case managers asked about the following issues:

What if the case manager did not think the client could handle their own care?
How will we stay informed about the client's health and problems with service?
Who will be monitoring their care?
What about the fear of abuse or exploitation from an employee?
What will happen to our jobs?

The first four of these questions reflect concern that self-directed consumers might not receive good care or appropriate monitoring if they (the consumers) were given too much responsibility. These case managers were worried about negative outcomes and about the fact that they might not be able to intervene appropriately to prevent or manage problems with care. These concerns illustrate well the beneficence versus maternalism struggle. The final issue regarding case manager jobs had two components: whether the new program was designed to cut case manager costs (assuming that case managers would spend less time with self-directed clients), and whether giving more responsibility and autonomy to clients would undermine the professional role of care management. As early volunteers for the program, these case managers were comfortable enough to be honest about their concerns; they were also invested in helping to get the new program off the ground. They worked through their concerns during the course of the discussion, concluding with the following comments:

> "CDC is the epitome of self-determination. As case managers, we are allowing our clients to make their own decisions, handle their own home care problems, and contact case managers at appropriate times."

> "We are trusting our clients to let us know when there is a problem, if they become overwhelmed, or have a change in health status."

> "We are first a trainer, then an observer."

> "The joy and personal satisfaction felt by case management staff in monitoring a client's health and homecare services becomes a joy in seeing her be the most independent person she can be."

As the demonstration got close to implementation, a training session for all case managers was arranged. The training occurred prior to any enrollment into consumer-directed services; before the training session began, participants completed a survey of their knowledge, attitudes, and opinions about consumer direction. All case managers within the program were expected to attend the training session, whether they were going to be involved with consumer-directed care or not. This decision to train all case managers on consumer self-direction reflected a commitment by agency leaders to promote awareness of the philosophy and practice of this new program option. Fifty case managers attended the training and completed the survey. These 50 participants covered the spectrum, including those who had indicated early interest in CDC, as well as those who had expressed serious reservations and did not want to work with self-directed clients.

Table 5.1 shows the results from this survey. Many case managers (45%) did not think they had a good understanding of consumer direction, although they appeared to know that CDC would be a shift away from traditional service provision. Just over 70% of case managers understood that case management in a CDC model would emphasize teaching and coaching. The overwhelming majority of case managers felt that it was good to give consumers more choice and control over how services are provided. Although the case managers agreed with the philosophy of more consumer choice and control, many (46%) questioned whether clients would want to manage their own services.

Would consumers' services be better? A high proportion (67%) of case managers were concerned about the quality of care, and about one-third said that they would worry more about their clients if they chose

Table 5.1 Case Manager Mean Responses and Percentage Agreeing
to Survey Items ($N = 50$)

	Mean	% Agree*
I have a good understanding of what consumer direction is.	2.49	55.1
Consumer direction gives clients more control over how they receive their services.	2.19	72.9
Case management with consumer direction clients emphasizes teaching and coaching.	2.18	71.1
There is a need for consumer direction in the ESP.	2.10	70.8
It is a good idea to give clients more say in how their services are delivered.	1.82	93.9
I am concerned that my clients' needs will not be adequately met under consumer direction.	2.63	50.0
I think consumer direction is the best way for some clients to receive services.	2.36	59.6
I feel comfortable recommending consumer direction to a client.	2.69	41.7
I am concerned about the quality of care for consumer-directed clients.	2.31	66.7
The benefits of consumer direction outweigh possible increased risks.	2.80	36.6
I think most ESP clients will not want to manage their own services.	2.67	45.8
I would worry more about my clients' well-being if they became consumer-directed.	2.91	32.6
I feel comfortable working with consumer-directed clients.	2.71	43.8

Note: Scale: 1 = strongly agree; 2 = agree; 3 = neutral; 4 = disagree; 5 = strongly disagree.
*Column shows percentage who agree or strongly agree.

self-direction. The choice and control that case managers believed consumers should have did *not* outweigh their concern about possible risks. About one in three case managers thought that the benefits offset the risks. Importantly, less than half felt comfortable working with self-directed clients or recommending the option based on what they knew.

The findings from this survey suggest that, prior to the start of a consumer-directed program, case managers were unequivocal about the importance of client autonomy and choice and understood that the case manager role would be different with self-directed clients. But they did not feel confident about their understanding of consumer direction, and they were concerned about risks and quality of care.

After the CDC program had been in place for about 10 months, we conducted focus groups with case managers to learn about their experiences working with clients who had chosen to self-direct their services.

Participants in the two focus groups were 24 case managers who were currently overseeing clients enrolled in the program. The focus groups took place at the end of August 2002. The 90-minute discussions were guided by questions regarding the impact of the CDC option on the consumer, on the current long-term care delivery system, and on the case management profession. Other issues emerged out of the conversations to illuminate case manager opinions, assessments, and feelings regarding the process and structure of the CDC initiative.

1. *What does consumer direction mean for the long-term care system, and for your clients?*

   The case managers highlighted several positive aspects of CDC for the consumer, including greater flexibility, more options, fewer complaints about workers, more hours of service for the same money, more trust in the workers, a greater comfort level with workers, better workers, more independence for consumers, more satisfaction, and a greater sense of role responsibility for both consumers and family members. Some case managers also mentioned an increase in well-being and self-esteem in the consumers. One discussion group participant mentioned that because the client finally had means to give something back to the person who was helping her and this reciprocity made her feel better. Another participant mentioned how a once difficult client has appeared to "have found his niche" and is currently very happy with services. Furthermore, some case managers felt that CDC could potentially serve clients better as a more culturally appropriate choice for diverse populations since clients choose their own workers and often hire family or friends—workers who know and understand them. Participants also mentioned that consumer direction appears to be a partial solution to labor shortages within home care agencies. Some case managers thought that the increased coverage (more services for the same cost) would reduce burnout for unpaid family caregivers.

   The question also elicited some negative opinions and attitudes about CDC in relationship to the family and the consumer. Several case managers wondered whether services were truly being delivered by family workers at a level of quality that would be considered acceptable under the traditional system. One case manager asked, "What if the client is happy and the worker is not doing a thing?" Other concerns included consumer difficulty in understanding the materials related to hiring workers and establishing payroll accounts, consumer unwillingness or inability to take on the responsibility of directing their own services, ideological issues about paying family members to do what might be considered their obligation, and concerns over motivations of family members. An extreme example of this latter concern was a client who admitted that she would like to hire a family member because the family member needed the money. Many of the concerns can be summarized with quotes from two of the case managers: "What is the right system of checks and balances, especially to find out if there are any changes with workers, with the client's health situation, with the client's needs?" and "How do you decide that the situation is so problematic that you need to do something about it?"

Finally, some case managers said that what really made CDC appropriate for a client or how it affected them really depended on the clients' unique characteristics and circumstances. For example, one case manager mentioned having a consumer that she was sure would succeed with self-direction but did not, whereas another case manager highlighted a case where a client truly enjoyed the new services but had been a difficult client in the traditional program.

2. *What is the impact of CDC on the case management profession?*

Responses to this question were many and varied, ranging from positive changes that might be fostered by consumer direction to concerns about the role of case management in the future. One case manager was sure that CDC would have no noticeable impact on the case management profession. Others responded that it was a very positive development, allowing for creative and flexible approaches to working with consumers based on their needs and abilities.

This question also elicited responses questioning the role of the case manager in relation to quality management and ongoing monitoring of services. There was a fair amount of consensus about the tension between "letting go" and continuing to provide professionally sound case management. Less contact with their clients was problematic for several of the case managers. How would they know if there was a problem or if the consumer's health situation changed in some way? Who would be liable? One specific example was the case of cognitive decline and its effects on care needs; case managers expressed concern about who would monitor those changes. Overall, there was a great deal of discussion about the ways in which consumer direction calls for something of a paradigm shift for case managers, and that perhaps there was not yet enough clarity or guidance to help in making that shift. All case managers stated their respect for the autonomy and preferences of every client, but several struggled with finding the right balance between professional intervention and empowerment-enhancing distance. Participants discussed the different kinds of roles and skills that come into play with self-directed clients, including teaching and coaching.

Other topics included the appropriate level of assistance with employment-related paperwork. Most consumers have some difficulty with all of the forms related to hiring their workers. Case managers were concerned about whether getting too involved in helping with paperwork was a departure from the ideals of consumer direction. One case manager offered the analogy of a real estate agent who tells home buyers where to sign at the closing of a sale; she suggested that the agent was providing a service, that no home buyer wants to become an expert on that particular type of paperwork; and that the assistance provided to self-directed clients with paperwork can be seen as a similar kind of service, and not as a threat to their independence and autonomy.

Finally, there was a great deal of agreement that consumer-directed participants do not necessarily require less case manager time than do traditional clients. The kinds of professional services that self-directed clients need might be different, but most case managers felt that CDC clients took as much time as traditional clients, especially at the beginning when they are going through training and paperwork for employing their workers.

3. *Based on your experiences in this pilot program, what aspects would you change or improve?*

Participants offered several suggestions about ways the program could be improved. Specific issues included consumer training, eligibility/appropriateness of participants for consumer direction, and changing expectations of case managers who are working with self-directed clients.

With respect to training consumers, one case manager said that the consumer manual included helpful information, but during the training sessions with consumers it became clear that the manual was not always well suited to the consumer's concerns and situation. Case managers generally agreed that the manual would need to be adapted to maximize its flexible use. Furthermore, there was a tendency for clients to not even follow it, leaving the case manager the task of walking them through the process from afar.

The topic of eligibility or appropriateness of clients for self-direction was an ongoing issue. There were concerns about who could, should, and would enroll in the CDC option. Case managers agreed that clearer guidelines about who could choose the program would be useful. An instrument that assessed an individual's skills and training needs would allow case managers to help consumers get what they needed to succeed in consumer direction. The instrument could also potentially help them decide who is allowed to be in the program.

Another continuing challenge was the changing and sometimes unclear role of case managers and the impact of this new program on caseload expectations. Case managers felt that it was essential for their supervisors to realize the complexities involved with implementing CDC. More time was being spent with CDC clients than originally assumed. Some specific concerns were highlighted. It appeared that there was an incomplete understanding of how exactly case management should be provided for consumer-directed clients. Case managers expressed a range of opinions about how best to provide support to the client. A specific example concerned the clients' formal level of care designation, which specifies a contact schedule (i.e., how frequently and in what form contact should be initiated by the case manager). This example speaks to concerns about not only giving the client autonomy and responsibility in self-directed care but also wanting to maintain some control over, and initiative in, contact with consumers. Other examples dealt with client's assessment (how often a self-directed client should be reassessed), the amount of time that should be spent with the client, and how much time should elapse between visits.

Time management for case managers was a real challenge as well. Case managers had been maintaining a traditional caseload of about 105 to 120 clients, in addition to taking on new CDC clients and providing their training. The CDC case managers were completing over 30 visits per month. With documentation requirements, administrative commitments, and the crises that invariably arise, case managers were extremely challenged in their efforts to remain on top of their workloads. In addition, the clients' two, 1-hour training sessions were not sufficient. Training has evolved into two, 2-hour sessions, along with phone calls, and additional visits to help with paperwork.

SUMMARY AND CONCLUSIONS

Some of the issues raised in the early discussions about the challenges of consumer direction for case managers were echoed throughout this demonstration project. The tension between commitment to greater client autonomy and worry about the client's well-being were heightened by the new CDC program. Results from the survey about case manager attitudes and knowledge of CD also reflected this tension. Focus groups with case managers that occurred after they had some experience with self-directed clients showed some alleviation of this worry. Before the program began, two-thirds of the case managers said that the benefits of consumer direction would not outweigh the risks to clients. After the option had been in place for several months, case managers were much more convinced about the benefits of consumer self-direction.

The focus groups also provided invaluable information about what it takes to implement a service approach as innovative as consumer direction. Case managers helped us to understand the distance that can exist between the "ideal," imagined, or philosophical version of a program and its actual implementation. Their discussion of the advantages and challenges of the program will provide guidance for the improvement of CDC at CoA and for other agencies that hope to put consumer direction into practice.

Case managers are an integral part of this program, and their evolving roles are perhaps the most challenging and central key to the success of the option. Even if only 10% of clients select this option, the new demands on case managers (i.e., helping with paperwork, taking on new roles such as educator and coach, and balancing consumer independence with professional standards) will continue to be a challenge. The overall goal for implementing CDC in this agency was to provide a continuum of service delivery options so that consumers can choose what is most appropriate for them. It is a significant paradigm shift for case managers to move among different roles and to use different priorities for consumers along this continuum of service delivery models. Certainly the same principles of professional practice underpin both approaches, but CDC pushes against existing boundaries regarding flexibility and client centeredness. The case managers in this research provided valuable insight about the challenges and benefits of making this shift.

ACKNOWLEDGMENTS

This project was supported in part by Council on Aging of Southwest Ohio. The authors would also like to acknowledge Tammie Hitt and Kristen Parker Wills for their work on this research.

REFERENCES

Applebaum, R. A., & Austin, C. (1990). *Long-term case management: Design and evaluation*. New York: Springer.

Geron, S. M. (2000). The quality of consumer-directed long-term care. *Generations*, 24(3), 66–73.

Infeld, D. L. (2004). *States' Experiences Implementing Consumer-Directed Home and Community Services: Results of the 2004 Survey of State Administrators, Opinion Survey and Telephone Interviews.* Washington, DC: National Association of State Units on Aging and The National Council on the Aging.

Kunkel, S. R., Duffy-Durham, L., & Scala, M. A. (2000). Consumer direction and traditional case management: Common ground or contested terrain? In R. Applebaum & M. White (Eds.), *Key issues in case management around the globe* (pp. 104–112). San Francisco, CA: American Society on Aging.

Micco, A., Hamilton, A. C. S., Martin, M. J., & McEwan, K. L. (1995). Case manager attitudes toward client-directed care. *Generations, 16,* 17–22.

Scala, M. A., & Mayberry, P. S. (1997). *Consumer-directed home services: Issues and models.* Oxford, OH: Scripps Gerontology Center.

Scala, M. A., Mayberry, P. S., & Kunkel, S. R. (1996). Consumer-directed home care: Client profiles and service challenges. *Journal of Case Management, 5*(3), 91–98.

Schneider, B. W., Mahoney, K. J., & Simon-Rusinowitz, L. (2001). *Encyclopedia of care of the elderly: Consumer directed care for the elderly.* Unpublished manuscript.

CHAPTER SIX

Integrating Occupational Health and Safety Into the United States' Personal Assistance Services Workforce Research Agenda

Teresa Scherzer
Susan Chapman
Robert Newcomer

INTRODUCTION

Occupational health researchers recognize that occupational injury is a prevalent problem in long-term care, including in-home services. However, there is a noticeable lack of research and policy attention to this problem among workers providing personal assistance services (PAS)— the personal care and housekeeping tasks that enable elderly and disabled persons to live in community settings. Occupational injury among these workers is thought to contribute to worker turnover, and in this way it may further exacerbate the growing problem of workforce recruitment and retention in this vital sector of long-term care. A further concern is that problems addressing occupational injury in PAS may increase as more of this assistance is obtained through consumer-directed models of care, in which PAS workers are "independent providers" hired, directed, and fired by individual PAS consumers.

Across the nation, PAS (also known as home care or in-home care) is a primary mode of long-term care, providing essential support such as bathing, dressing, and grocery shopping for people with disabilities who live in community settings. This workforce has nearly doubled over the past 10 years, from 500,000 to more than 1 million workers nationally (Kaye, Chapman, Newcomer, & Harrington, 2005). Census Bureau estimates place the number at 1.2 million in 2003 (U.S. Census Bureau, 2003). The expansion of PAS is due to multiple factors: the aging of the population, PAS's presumed cost-effectiveness, the preference of persons to remain in community settings, and State compliance with the Supreme Court's ruling in the 1999 *Olmstead* case. A major feature of this expansion is the increasing diffusion of consumer-directed models of service delivery. This topic is covered in depth elsewhere in this book.

The central role of PAS and the increasing presence of consumer direction, however, are accompanied by what some have characterized as an unfolding crisis of labor supply. The number of persons needing PAS is projected to increase through 2025, while at the same time the numbers of paraprofessionals are expected to fall short of the projected service demand (Summer, Friedland, Mack, & Mathieu, 2004). One response to these trends is that, since 2001, public and private sector resources have funded over 100 state and local projects that attempt to increase the labor supply. These incorporate various strategies, among which are improving worker retention through increased wages, benefits, training, mentoring, career ladders, and worker associations (Scherzer, Chapman, & Newcomer, 2004).

Decreasing PAS's long-standing problem of high worker turnover (i.e., short duration of employment) is one key to maintaining or bolstering its labor supply. Turnover is attributed to a combination of low wages, lack of benefits, the often variable working hours, and the physical and emotional difficulty of the work. Another factor—discussed much less often than the others—is the role of occupational injury.

This chapter has three purposes. The first is to review what is known about occupational injury in PAS. Next, we discuss how the growth of consumer direction in PAS may offer both opportunities and obstacles for addressing occupational injury. We conclude by discussing the implications of integrating occupational health and safety into the larger PAS workforce agenda.

OCCUPATIONAL INJURY IN HOME CARE

Most of the research about occupational injury among home care workers is from Scandinavia, including several population-based studies (Broberg,

1993, cited in Johansson, 1995; Brulin, Winkvist, & Langendoen, 2000; Dellve, Lagerstrom, & Hagberg, 2002, 2003; Johansson, 1995; Malker et al., 1990, cited in Johansson, 1995; Ono, Lagerstrom, Hagberg, Linden, & Malker, 1995; Swedish National Board of Occupational Safety and Health, 1991, cited in Johansson, 1995). Studies of Swedish home care workers show that, compared to the female working population at large, and specific occupational groups, they have significantly higher rates of work-related musculoskeletal disorders (WRMSDs; sprains, strains, tears, soreness, pain, and other disorders caused by overuse or misuse of muscles, tendons, nerves; overexertion; and by extreme or repetitive bending or twisting) and overexertion injuries (e.g., an injury caused by lifting something that is too heavy for one's capacity; Johansson; Ono et al.). For example, Ono and colleagues found that the annual injury incidence rates from overexertion accidents and WRMSDs were 19.2 and 15.1 per 1,000 workers, respectively. The main risk factor for home care worker injury was handling the client (e.g., transferring and assistance with dressing and ambulation)—particularly lifting (81% of all reported injuries). Psychosocial stress is also thought to combine with physical workload to increase the risk of injury (Dellve et al., 2003; Johansson).

WRMSDs are the most frequently cited causes for work-related injury and days lost from work (Ono et al., 1995). Ono and colleagues found that the mean duration of sick leave among home care workers due to overexertion accidents was 3.5 days, and 101.6 days for WRMSDs. The total lost work time due to sick leave from these two types of injury accounted for about 8.2% of all work-related sick days among all employed persons in Sweden in 1990 to 1991, although home care workers constitute about 5% of the working population.

In contrast to the Scandinavian research, which has been specific to home care workers, studies of the direct care workforce in the United States have often not differentiated home care workers from institutional care workers. One of the few studies specifically on U.S. home care (PAS) workers was conducted in 1990 in Washington state, in which 1,900 home care workers from 16 agencies were surveyed about working conditions (Hayashi, Gibson, & Weatherley, 1994). Hayashi and colleagues found working conditions to be poor, with low pay and few benefits; unpaid overtime, training, and travel time; unstable schedules; and physically and emotionally stressful work, although many workers said they found the work itself satisfying. The study also found that almost 40% of respondents had experienced a work-related injury or health problem (including muscle strain and emotional stress), and 26% reported experiencing discrimination, harassment, or abuse on the job, especially verbal abuse (Hayashi et al.).

The major information source about paid workers and work injury is an annual survey of employers conducted by the Bureau of Labor Statistics (BLS) of the U.S. Department of Labor. With respect to PAS workers, there have been two substantial limitations in the BLS data. First, PAS workers have not been identifiable in data reported to the BLS. Instead, injury data are available for a broader grouping of related occupations (nursing aides, orderlies, and attendants) and home health care workers.[1] Importantly, too, the BLS survey data are obtained from employers—hospitals, nursing homes, and home health care agencies. Consequently, even with a better delineation of PAS workers from other types of direct care paraprofessionals, PAS workers employed in consumer-directed services (i.e., as "independent providers" who do not work for organizations or agencies) are excluded from the sample frame. Estimates of the number of independent providers in the PAS workforce vary depending on the data source. National surveys such as the Current Population Survey place the estimate of independent PAS workers to be 8.9% nationally (Kaye, Chapman, Newcomer, & Harrington, 2005). However, state administrative records show much higher rates. For example, in California, approximately 80% of the 300,000 PAS workers are independent providers (Scherzer, Kang, Chapman, & Newcomer, 2005).

Recognizing the limitations in the BLS survey, it is nevertheless noteworthy that the findings show that the occupational category "nursing aides, orderlies, and attendants" had 79,000 occupation injuries severe enough to cause at least 1 day of missed work in 2002. This was second only to the 112,000 injuries of truck drivers (Bureau of Labor Statistics, 2004). Most of these injured direct care workers (56%) suffered sprains and strains to the trunk (usually the back), likely related to lifting or moving residents. The median number of days away from work was 6, but 18.5% of these direct care workers missed 1 month or more (BLS).

Studies that have attempted to look more specifically at home-based workers have largely focused on home health care workers (HHCWs; BLS, 1997; Galinsky, Waters, & Malit, 2001; Meyer & Muntaner, 1999; Myers, Jensen, Nestor, & Rattiner, 1993). Statistics relative to HHCWs are informative because home health care and PAS workers share some of the same occupational risks, some of which include working in private homes which often involves patient handling. Both HHCWs and PAS workers usually work alone—without direct supervision and without assistance from coworkers; and usually work without the lifts, other

---

[1] However, changes in survey methodology are expected to make data on PAS workers available in Spring 2005 (Personal communication, Occupational Safety and Health staff email, February 18, 2005).

assistive devices, or adjustable furniture that are common to hospitals or nursing homes, and which can prevent injury to both workers and consumers (BLS; Galinsky et al.; Meyer & Muntaner; Myers et al.). However, there are also important differences. Among these, most HHCWs are employed by agencies, conduct some medical tasks, and have access to task training. Occupational injury and days lost from work are prevalent among HHCWs. For example, BLS data show that the injury rate for HHCWs was about 50% higher than that of hospital workers (474 vs. 326 cases per 10,000 full-time employees [FTE]). The rate of overexertion injuries among HHCWs was 183/10,000 FTE, compared to 144/10,000 FTE in hospitals (BLS). Of the overexertion injuries experienced by HHCWs, more than half were from lifting clients.

In another study, Meyer and Muntaner (1999) compared workers' compensation claims for occupational injury and disability of HHCWs, nursing home workers, and hospital-based workers. Annual incidence of injury for HHCWs was 52 per 1,000 workers, a rate lower than that of nursing home workers (132/1,000), but higher than that of hospital workers (46/1,000). Mean number of days away from work was significantly higher for HHCWs (44), compared to 18 for nursing home workers and 14 for hospital workers. These rates suggest that injuries filed for workers' compensation may be more severe and disabling among home-based workers. Whether this extends to all occupational injuries has not been as well documented.

Another frequent cause of occupational injury among HHCWs is motor vehicle accidents (BLS, 1997; Meyer & Muntaner, 1999). Meyer and Muntaner found this to have caused 14% of all injuries, following falls (16%) and overexertion (47%). These accidents are occupational injuries because they are sustained when workers drive from one client's home to another (injuries sustained while commuting at the beginning and end of the workday are not counted as occupational injuries). This risk is also thought to be common among PAS workers, who are frequently assigned to two or more clients per day (Hayashi, Gibson, & Weatherley, 1994).

CONSUMER DIRECTION AND
PAS OCCUPATIONAL SAFETY

Consumer direction among persons with disabilities has resulted in at least two major changes for the PAS workforce. These are expected to have an impact on occupational safety and injury. First, consumer direction has changed the relationship between workers and recipients. PAS workers under this model are "independent providers." They are directly hired and fired by individuals, not by an agency. Training, which has never been a strong component of home care workforce development, is now often delegated to the consumer. Second, an increasing percentage of paid PAS workers are related to consumers. In California's In-Home Supportive Services (IHSS) program, the oldest and most developed consumer-directed model of PAS in the United States, approximately 52% of workers are related to the consumers for whom they provide care (Scherzer et al., 2005). In addition, a majority of participants in all three Cash and Counseling demonstration programs (New York, Arkansas, and Florida) chose family providers as their paid PAS workers (Dale, Brown, Phillips, & Carlson, 2003; Doty, 2004).

Consumer direction may offer both opportunities and obstacles for addressing occupational risk and injury. Does the use of family providers help to reduce occupational hazards in the home, or are worker and consumer injuries less likely to be reported? Are family providers more or less willing to provide whatever assistance is required by their elderly or disabled family members regardless of their experience or ability to perform these tasks? Are family providers more aware than nonrelatives of environmental risks like throw rugs, slippery floors, and unstable furniture? Are they in a better situation for changing these risk situations?

With regard to occupational health and safety, does the use of consumer-directed services result in unintended difficulties and obstacles for addressing occupational hazards and injury (regardless of the consumer-provider relationship)? In consumer-directed models there may be potential ambiguities about who is responsible for addressing risks, providing liability insurance (i.e., workers' compensation), and addressing claims reporting and assistance for injured workers. Unlike the agency model of PAS, consumer direction does not have a traditional "management" that instructs workers about their rights to a safe workplace and to workers' compensation benefits, and to which workers may report occupational hazards or injury. Moreover, consumer-directed models might not have systems for backup coverage to replace an injured or ill worker, or even sick day benefits. All of this may unintentionally lead workers to work while injured or delay seeking medical attention.

Delayed medical attention for work injuries, the underreporting of injuries, and the delay or denial of workers' compensation claims may have serious consequences for independent providers' health and ability to work as needed by the consumers. The burden of occupational injury on PAS consumers may mean that they will have to seek out, hire, and train a new worker. For disabled persons receiving care at home, the need to repeatedly train new workers for their specific care may be stressful and time-consuming. These issues are in addition to anxiety over whether workers will be reliable in showing up for work and their willingness and ability to do what is needed (Foster, Brown, Phillips, & Carlson, 2003).

An example of the potential adverse consequences on PAS worker health is from a recent study by investigators from the National Institute for Occupational Safety and Health (NIOSH, 2004) that specifically examined the risk of occupational injury and working conditions among independent providers or consumer-directed PAS workers. This study included multilingual focus groups with PAS workers, key informant interviews, analysis of injury data, and an in-home site visit. The study found that housekeeping tasks were as physically demanding as client handling, few workers had adequate tools or equipment for their required work tasks, most consumers' homes were not equipped so that services could be provided effectively or safely, and most PAS workers lacked previous training and opportunities for future training on how to safely conduct PAS work. Several of these issues were also noted in earlier studies (Hayashi et al., 1994; Ono et al., 1995). The investigators concluded that the then-current arrangements of consumer-directed PAS "could lead to health and safety problems for home care [PAS] workers. Lack of training, inadequate resources, and poor communication between consumers and caregivers contributed to these health risks" (NIOSH, 2004).

Another dimension of this NIOSH (2004) study included an examination of workers' compensation claims by IHSS workers. During the period January through October 2001, there were 17 claims by PAS workers—from among approximately 12,000 IHSS workers in the study county. This low incidence contrasted sharply with focus group data that showed that many PAS workers experienced "pain" or "lots of pain" in the back, neck, shoulders, and lower extremities at the end of a typical workday. The underuse of worker's compensation was suggested as resulting from a lack of knowledge of workers' compensation, and lack of backup coverage for the PAS worker. Few of the interviewed IHSS workers were aware of their rights under workers' compensation. Instead, they frequently paid out of pocket for medical treatment or alternative therapies (e.g., healing ointments and community healers). Moreover, many workers said they "could not afford to miss work" because the time off would be unpaid and because the consumer would be without help (NIOSH). The NIOSH study results are nearly identical to preliminary findings from a research study (in progress) by the first author, based on in-depth interviews with independent providers who had an occupational injury.

Occupational risk and injury have been addressed somewhat in research comparing the experiences of participants and workers in agency and consumer-directed models (Benjamin & Matthias, 2004; Dale et al., 2003); however, the emphasis of the work has been on stress and satisfaction. Benjamin and Matthias compared agency-employed and consumer-directed workers on six measures of stress and four measures of satisfaction. Worker experience and outcomes varied, but on most measures, consumer-directed workers had the same or better outcomes compared to agency-employed workers. Occupational risk and injury was not explicitly addressed, although two of the six stress measures imply some injury risk: Recipient Behavior (recipient yells or threatens worker; measure also includes "hazards of work") and Recipient Role (clarity about roles for recipient and worker). Investigators found that when they controlled for worker and recipient characteristics and working conditions, the consumer-directed model was associated with better outcomes on Relationship with Recipient (being clear and comfortable with consumer's authority) and Recipient Role. Worker stress on Recipient Behavior did not differ significantly between agency- and consumer-directed models. Family workers had better outcomes on Relationship with Recipient compared to nonfamily workers, indicating the shared interests between consumers and family providers (Benjamin & Matthias; Doty, 2004).

One study comparing agency workers and independent providers has explicitly measured the occurrence of occupational injury. This exception is the evaluation of a Cash and Counseling demonstration program known as Arkansas' Independent Choices. Dale and colleagues (2003) found that when differences in total hours of care provided were accounted for, consumer-directed workers were no more likely than agency workers to experience work-related physical injury or strain. Family members accounted for 78% of the independent providers in the Arkansas program.

INTEGRATING OCCUPATIONAL HEALTH AND SAFETY INTO THE PAS WORKFORCE AGENDA

The occupational risks in PAS, the changes in PAS due to the expansion of consumer direction, and the current limitations in data systems documenting occupational injury are important policy issues within the field of long-term care.

Over the short term, one challenge will be how to address the risk of occupational injury in PAS and balance worker safety with consumers' control over their supportive services. Another challenge emerging from consumer direction is the new employment situation for workers and consumers. Although consumer direction empowers the consumer, it may unintentionally disadvantage workers if there are no clear avenues for addressing occupational hazards and injury, as well as other concerns such as an payroll mistakes or worker–consumer conflict. Moreover, although recent research finds that consumers and known/related workers generally report greater satisfaction with consumer-directed models than with agency models, and possibly better health outcomes (Benjamin & Matthias, 2004; Doty, 2004), it is unknown how these close personal relationships will influence consumers' or workers' willingness to identify and address potential occupational hazards, report injury, or file a workers' compensation claim.

Various organizational infrastructures have begun to emerge to help enable consumer-directed models. One of the most visible and important developments is the widespread use by state consumer-directed programs of Financial Management Services (FMS), which primarily assist consumers with employer-related fiscal management (e.g., payroll and tax withholding for PAS workers). Other developments include the development of provider registries (that may screen potential providers and facilitate consumer-worker matches), and consumer training and case management (that provide assistance to consumers about managing PAS-related budgets, and hiring, training, and firing workers).

Concerns about worker safety in consumer direction have lagged behind these other developments. However, in certain regions of the country, labor unions have markedly improved working conditions for independent providers by helping to establish Employers of Record, an entity that expands the role of FMS by establishing legal employment relationships with an aggregate workforce of independent providers. With an Employer of Record, workers may unionize and collectively bargain for improved working conditions—including health and safety training, health benefits (including specifics about eligibility and share of monthly premiums), and access to workers' compensation. These important gains for PAS workers, however, are unevenly distributed throughout the country and do not reflect the general work situation in PAS (Hayashi et al., 1994; Heinritz-Canterbury, 2002). In terms of worker occupational safety and health during the continued expansion of consumer direction, it will be important to systematically educate workers and consumers about who is responsible for which tasks, including addressing occupational hazards and filing a workers' compensation claim. The active role of a third party or parties, such as labor unions or Employers of Record, may be critical to address these issues because of the ability to reach all consumers and workers on a system-wide level.

In our review of the home care/PAS literature, we found few studies that focused on working conditions and occupational risk and no studies that examined the effect of provider or consumer training on occupational risk or injury, or the consequences of occupational injury. Limitations in the U.S. data systems pose serious barriers to examining prevalence, incidence, correlates, and consequences of occupational injury in PAS. These limitations also preclude analyses of the effects of occupational injury on worker turnover and worker and consumer well-being. Establishing new data systems that take into account the changing environment of PAS could be a crucial first step in meeting this challenge.

Protecting the health and safety of PAS workers appears to be a formidable challenge—but there are numerous opportunities for meeting this challenge. Every PAS program across the county is a potential laboratory for exploring the causes of and solutions to occupational injury. In the context of the continued expansion of consumer-directed PAS, and the increasing demand for workers, this may be the appropriate time for a more systematic effort to compile and exchange information on program models and their outcomes, and build conceptual and practical bridges between the domains of PAS workforce research and occupational health and safety. Integrating occupational safety and health into the PAS workforce research agenda may provide new answers to the problem of worker turnover, and new ways to forge lasting linkages between quality jobs and quality care.

REFERENCES

Benjamin, A. E., & Matthias, R. E. (2004). Work-life differences and outcomes for agency and consumer-directed home-care workers. *Gerontologist, 44*(4), 479–488.

Brulin, C., Winkvist, A., & Langendoen, S. (2000). Stress from working conditions among home care personnel with musculoskeletal symptoms. *Journal of Advanced Nursing, 31*(1), 181–189.

Bureau of Labor Statistics. (1997). *Injuries to caregivers working in patients' homes (Summary 97-4)*. Washington, DC: U.S. Department of Labor.

Bureau of Labor Statistics. (2004). *Lost-worktime injuries and illnesses: Characteristics and resulting days away from work, 2002 (News Release)*: U.S. Department of Labor.

Dale, S., Brown, R., Phillips, B., & Carlson, B. (2003). *The experiences of workers hired under consumer direction in Arkansas* (No. 8349-105). Princeton, NJ: Mathematica Policy Research, Inc.

Dellve, L., Lagerstrom, M., & Hagberg, M. (2002). Rehabilitation of home care workers: Supportive factors and obstacles prior to disability pension due to musculoskeletal disorders. *Journal of Occupational Rehabilitation, 12*(2), 55–64.

Dellve, L., Lagerstrom, M., & Hagberg, M. (2003). Work-system risk factors for permanent work disability among home-care workers: A case-control study. *International Archives of Occupational and Environmental Health, 76*(3), 216–224.

Doty, P. (2004). *Consumer-directed home care: effects on family caregivers*. San Francisco, CA: Family Caregiver Alliance.

Foster, L., Brown, R., Phillips, B., & Carlson, B. L. (2003). *Easing the burden of caregiving: The impact of consumer-direction on primary informal caregivers in Arkansas (Final Report)*. Princeton, NJ: Mathematica Policy Research, Inc.

Galinsky, T., Waters, T., & Malit, B. (2001). Overexertion injuries in home health care workers and the need for ergonomics. *Home Health Care Services Quarterly, 20*(3), 57–73.

Hayashi, R., Gibson, J. W., & Weatherley, R. A. (1994). Working conditions in home care: a survey of Washington state's home care workers. *Home Health Care Services Quarterly, 14*(4), 37–48.

Heinritz-Canterbury, J. (2002). *Collaborating to improve in-home supportive services: stakeholder perspectives on implementing California's public authorities*. Bronx, NY: Paraprofessional Healthcare Institute.

Johansson, J. A. (1995). Psychosocial work factors, physical work load and associated musculoskeletal symptoms among home care workers. *Scandinavian Journal of Psychology, 36*, 113–129.

Kaye, H. S., Chapman, S., Newcomer, R., & Harrington, C. (2005). Rapid expansion of the home- and community-based personal assistance workforce (PAS Working Paper).

Meyer, J. D., & Muntaner, C. (1999). Injuries in home health care workers: An analysis of occupational morbidity from a state compensation database. *American Journal of Industrial Medicine, 35*(3), 295–301.

Myers, A., Jensen, R. C., Nestor, D., & Rattiner, J. (1993). Low back injuries among home health aides compared with hospital nursing aides. *Home Health Care Services Quarterly, 14*(2/3), 149–155.

National Institute for Occupational Safety and Health. (2004). *NIOSH health hazard evaluation report: Alameda County Public Authority for in-home support services*. Cincinnati, OH: National Institute for Occupational Safety and Health.

Ono, Y., Lagerstrom, M., Hagberg, M., Linden, A., & Malker, B. (1995). Reports of work related musculoskeletal injury among home care service workers compared with nursery school workers and the general population of employed women in Sweden. *Occupational and Environmental Medicine, 52*, 686–693.

Scherzer, T., Chapman, S., & Newcomer, R. (2004). *Workforce development projects in personal assistance services*. Retrieved January 8, 2005, from www.pascenter.org.

Scherzer, T., Kang, T., Chapman, S., & Newcomer, R. (2005). Factors associated with use of family providers in California's IHSS program, 2003 (PAS Working Paper).

Summer, L., Friedland, R., Mack, K., & Mathieu, S. (2004). *Measuring the years: state aging trends and indicators*. Washington, D.C.: Center on an Aging Society Health Policy Institute, Georgetown University, for the National Governors Association Center for Best Practices.

U.S. Census Bureau. (2003). *American community survey. Tabulations of public use microdata*. Retrieved March 2, 2005, from www.census.gov/acs/www/index.html.

CHAPTER SEVEN

Backs to the Future:

The Challenge of Individual Long-Term Care Planning

Kathryn B. McGrew

Consumer direction empowers individuals and families in a long-term care crisis to make meaningful decisions with expanded options and to exercise control over the care experience. Even though the various consumer-direction models have intuitive appeal, it has been a challenge to realize it in both policy and practice. We are now seeing empirical evidence that choice and control in long-term care increases satisfaction with care (Foster, Brown, Phillips, Schore, & Carlson, 2003), as well as anecdotal evidence that these forms of empowerment reduce the risk of institutionalization. Choice and control can be enhanced even further when individuals and families engage in planning well in advance of a long-term care crisis. With long-term care planning, consumer direction begins early. Planning expands care options by making decisions today for the eventuality of a long-term care need. Long-term care planning involves financial, social (including legal), and environmental (housing and living arrangement) decisions, within the means of individuals and families. When individuals and families engage in long-term care planning they may increase their power to purchase care, form agreements or understandings about family roles and responsibilities, and improve the accessibility of their home environments. When a long-term care need arises without long-term care planning, individuals and families are necessarily limited by the options before them.

Individual and family decisions about long-term care are usually made in a crisis, with insufficient plans and resources in place. The risks of limited options include reduced satisfaction with care, premature use of formal services (both institutional and home- and community-based), and diminished quality of life.

We are compelled to address this issue by six converging forces in long-term care policy and practice: (1) increasing demand for home and community-based services in supporting care at home, (2) escalating nursing home costs, (3) intense budget pressures related to Medicare and Medicaid, (4) a growing recognition of the value of consumer choice and consumer direction in long-term care, (5) a widening range of planning options such as advance directives and long-term care insurance, and (6) an aging population.

By encouraging and facilitating long-term care planning (in effect to promote individual engagement in early consumer direction), can we expand the choices available to individuals and their families, well before a need arises? Recent literature about long-term care planning suggests a broad range of obstacles to planning, from the reluctance of people to consider their own risk of dependency (Cutler, 1996; George, 1993; San Antonio & Rubenstein, 2004; Sörensen & Zarit, 1996) to the ambiguous messages about responsibility for long-term care (Kaiser Family Foundation, 2001; Mebane, 2001; Sörensen & Pinquart, 2000), to the lack of information for informed planning (Harvard School of Public Health and Louis Harris & Associates, 1996; Greenwald, M., & Associates, 1999).

In 1995, the Ohio Department of Aging introduced a long-term care consultation service called CareChoice Ohio. Its purpose was to provide an early intervention to assist people with long-term care planning before a nursing facility admission was requested. A weak response to this voluntary program prompted a focus group study, which was conducted for the state of Ohio to explore the dynamics of individual and family long-term care planning (or failure to plan). This project uses data from this focus group study.

METHODOLOGY

We designed focus group interviews to explore values, knowledge, and circumstances that drive planning or non-planning, as well as to identify key actors in the planning process. The objective was to address two broad questions. (1) What is the most effective way to reach prospective consumers in order to encourage and facilitate long-term care planning?

(2) What do prospective consumers need to make a comprehensive long-term care plan? This chapter explores the latter of the two original objectives.

The focus group is a tool designed to elicit group interaction around a set of questions or areas of interest. Participants are encouraged to share their individual stories, experiences, and ideas, and to respond to those of others. Although the groups examine specific areas of interest, other relevant issues may also emerge.

In a purposive sampling process, the researchers recruited participants for five focus groups across the state of Ohio, with a total of 43 participants.

The Insured (10 participants) were older adults who had engaged in financial planning such as purchasing long-term care insurance, reserving sufficient financial assets for potential long-term care expenses (self-insurance), or moving into a continuing care retirement community (CCRC), which provides a range of living options from independent living through skilled nursing care.

CareChoice Ohio (CCO) Clients (8 participants) had each received a CCO consultation.

Nursing Home Residents (6 participants) had moved into a nursing home without having engaged in any significant pre-admission planning behaviors.

Mixed Group (9 participants) were older adults recruited with a criterion of exclusion: none had purchased long-term care insurance, was self-insured, or had moved into a CCRC. These participants represented a range of planning behaviors, from none to limited long-term care planning, such as having made housing modifications.

Adult Children (10 participants) were adult children of older adults who received some form of long-term care services or who were at risk of needing long-term care services because of their extreme age. In the exploration of planning attitudes and behaviors, adult children were treated in this study as older adults themselves (average age 59), as well as proxies for their parents.

The researchers audiotaped and transcribed the focus group proceedings verbatim. Using procedures developed by Anselm Strauss (1987), the researchers analyzed the interview texts and conceptualized data in a developmental process of coding and categorizing. Findings led to the development of a conceptual model identifying dynamics and conditions essential to the pursuit of long-term care planning.

FINDINGS

Why do so many individuals and families arrive at a long-term care crisis with their backs to the future? This study suggests that pre-crisis planning for long-term care will occur only when a set of conditions is fully met. The conditions are necessary to move people from a state of inertia regarding long-term care, to the activities of pre-planning, to a planning decision or strategy. The model identifying these conditions and their relationship is found in Figure 7.1. The order of the conditions can be regarded as a stepwise path to long-term care planning; if any one of the conditions is not met along this path, the individual is unlikely to engage in long-term care planning.

The first condition is the Perception of Vulnerability or a sense that the issue of long-term care needs is potentially, personally relevant. *Could dependency happen to me?* The second condition is Perception of Timeliness, or the conclusion that personal vulnerability to future long-term care needs is an issue now. *Should I concern myself yet?* The third condition, Perception of Responsibility, is the value that the burden of responsibility for future care is, at least in part, one's own. *Whose responsibility is this?* The fourth condition, Perception of Control, is the belief that assuming responsibility for long-term care is within one's own control, not within the control of fate or powerful others. *Who has control?*

A positive response to the first two questions and a claim of personal responsibility and control in response to the third and fourth questions lead to the pre-planning phase, characterized by information gathering, inventory taking, and ultimately, decision making. The fifth condition, Adequacy of Information, is characterized by having enough accurate information about options, policies, programs, costs, and eligibility requirements to make informed decisions. *Do I have the needed information?* The sixth condition, Perception of Resources, is the sense that, given one's understanding of the options, programs, and eligibility requirements, one has sufficient material or social resources to commit to a long-term care plan. *Do I have the needed resources?*

The seventh and final condition, Rational Decision, is the calculated choice one makes now to invest time and resources toward an unpredictable future. The significance of the seventh condition is that even when all preceding conditions are met, individuals may make the decision not to commit to a plan and therefore to risk facing the need for long-term care without a plan in place. *Do I choose to invest resources now toward an unpredictable future?* An individual who chooses to plan may commit to a financial plan, a social/environmental plan, or, optimally, a comprehensive plan combining financial and other planning. See Areas of Planning for descriptions of these types of plans. The "end" of the path to

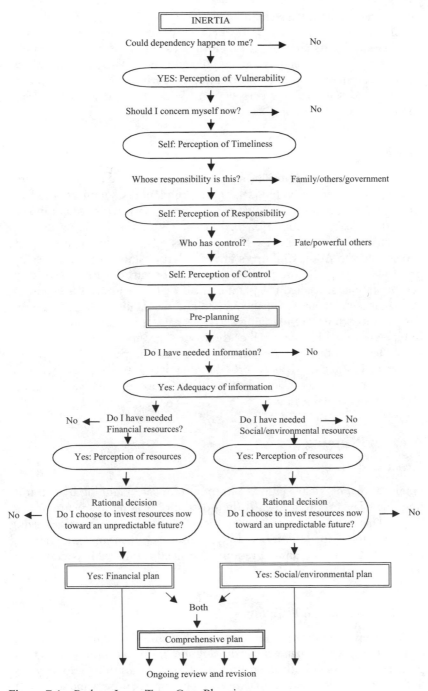

Figure 7.1   Path to Long-Term Care Planning.

long-term care planning is not a fixed place: the plan (or the risk) requires ongoing review and may require revision. Policies, programs, and eligibility requirements change, as do informal support systems. Individual health status and personal resources change as well. These changes necessitate a continual process of information gathering and inventory taking and may result in evolving perspectives about planning and risk-taking, and thus a modified plan.

Planner Types

Related to the seven conditions for planning, four broad types of planners emerged from this study: Non-planners, Pre-planners, Planners, and Risk Choosers. Non-planners are either in a state of inertia or have not moved beyond the first four conditions. Although all nursing home residents in this study are Non-planners, Non-planners are also found in both the Mixed and the Adult Children's groups. Participants who *have* met the first four criteria and are in the phase of information gathering and inventory taking are called Pre-planners. All CCO clients are Pre-planners, as well as some members of the Mixed and the Adult Children's groups. Participants whose pre-planning activities have led to a rational decision to plan are called Planners. All of the Insured groups are Planners, as are a few members of both the Mixed group and the parents of the Adult Children. Participants whose pre-planning activities have resulted in a decision not to take action are called Risk Choosers. Risk Choosers are found in the Mixed group.

Areas of Planning

Financial

Financial planners have engaged in long-term care planning by committing financial resources toward the possibility of long-term care dependency. This includes the purchase of long-term care insurance, reserving sufficient assets for long-term care expenses (self-insurance), or moving into a CCRC. Such planning requires financial resources beyond the capacity of many individuals.

Social/Environmental Planning

A social/environmental plan includes changing or adapting housing; changing living arrangements; shoring up informal support systems; preparing for crises with good information about options and services; and providing clear communication, including legal agreements, about health care preferences and wishes. This type of plan does not provide complete protection against the consequences of long-term care dependency and is regarded as a limited plan.

Comprehensive Planning

A combination of financial and social/environmental planning contributes to a comprehensive plan that provides maximum protection against the consequences of long-term care dependency. An effective comprehensive plan must be supported by sufficient material and social resources for its implementation. Although the perception of sufficient resources is necessary to *initiate* planning, sufficient *actual* resources are required to operationalize and sustain the plan.

Decisions about long-term care are seldom made in isolation. Discussions and/or negotiations between husband and wife or with adult children are evident in every stage along the planning path. The role of adult children in the planning and provision of long-term care is significant. This role was further explored in the focus group of Adult Children, and the influence of adult children was apparent in each of the conditions necessary for long-term care planning.

To promote and facilitate planning through policies, programs, and practices,we must understand the perceptions, needs, and experiences that encourage or discourage planning. What makes a Planner? A Nonplanner? A Risk Chooser? As is demonstrated in the following discussion, there was much variability among focus group participants in perceptions and behaviors regarding planning for long-term care. Non-planners, Preplanners, Planners, and Risk Choosers reflected both shared and different values and experiences in confronting the conditions along the planning path.

MOVING AWAY FROM INERTIA

Perception of Vulnerability: *Could dependency happen to me?*

Perceiving that one might need long-term care is necessary to begin planning. Without a perception of personal relevance, ideas, and information about long-term care—even scare tactics—are regarded, if attended to at all, as stories about *others*. Although not all focus group participants demonstrated a sense of vulnerability to long-term care *dependency,* nearly all acknowledged their own *mortality.* Indeed, when it came to planning behaviors, the majority of participants in all groups, with the exception of nursing home residents, described detailed plans for burials and cremations. Many had purchased cemetery lots, caskets, and head-stones already engraved with their names. A few had written their own obituaries. Several participants joked that they had planned everything for their deaths but the dates.

In contrast to this acknowledgment of mortality, several Non-planners expressed "never thinking" about the possibility that they might be vulnerable to long-term care dependency in late life. This is particularly true for the nursing home residents whose need for long-term care took them by surprise.

The good health, active lifestyles, and histories of family longevity of some of the Non-planners appear to contribute to a sense of invulnera-bility to dependency, or at least a rationale for postponing thinking about it. In the case of Planners, such a family history may trigger recognition that long life may bring problems.

For other Non-planners, surviving a health crisis appeared to con-tribute to a special sense of strength. And, for some, good health behaviors are perceived as a way of staving off a crisis. Many Non-planners told stories of the experiences of vulnerable others without translating these stories into warnings of personal vulnerability.

It is clear that there are many factors that contribute to a failure to see oneself as vulnerable; without such a sense an individual will remain a Non-planner. Planners and Pre-planners, in contrast, demonstrated a variety of factors that contributed to their sense of personal vulnerability. A clear sense of vulnerability may reflect an age consciousness developed from body cues, changes in health, or the experiences of others.

Those who do not consider the possibility of dependency or who feel invulnerable to it remain in a state of inertia regarding long-term care planning. Those who ask the question, Am I vulnerable to dependency? may also ask, What are the potential consequences to me of long-term care dependency? What are the costs to my family, my assets, and my fu-ture autonomy? It is these costs that will be weighed and calculated in the seventh and final step (Rational Decision) on the path toward long-term care planning. Pondering potential costs at the first (Perception of Vul-nerability) and second (Perception of Timeliness) stages is more a matter of imagination than calculation. Even so, imagining the impact of depen-dency may have an effect on the outcome of the second stage, Perception of Timeliness.

Perception of Timeliness: *Should I concern myself yet?*

Even when people have a sense of personal vulnerability to long-term care dependency, it does not follow that they will engage in pre-planning behaviors. This requires a perception that active thinking about the future is appropriate and called for, *now*. It is clear that there is no age deter-minant of timeliness. The oldest participant in the study, nearly 85 years old, had recently decided it was time to "plan ahead." In contrast, one of the younger participants, age 66, had already purchased long-term care insurance. Many had a sense that a time for serious thinking would come, but were vague about when that might happen.

> *"It's too far down the road for me. I don't even think about it"; "[It seems] all in the distance ... and I'm very much a NOW person, not a future person."*

One Non-planner argued that the possibility of a change in his per-spective by the time he needed care would render any decisions made today unreliable. Unable to anticipate his future circumstances, he felt unready to commit to pre-planning today:

> *"Well, I'm 68 and, uh, today I can hook up my six-thousand-pound travel trailer and haul it across the country, I feel real proud of the fact ... We travel, I bowl, I use all kinds of power tools ... Uh, maybe ten years from now I won't be able to do that. My thinking then will be entirely different from what it is now, I know. I could talk about [long-term care], but my feelings now would not necessarily be the same as they would be when I needed it. My attitude would be entirely different when I'm no longer able to do all this."*

Adult children can reinforce a state of inertia by their reluctance or refusal to engage in discussions about their parents' vulnerability or mortality. Some participants were given messages by children that such concerns were premature.

> *"[My children] will say, 'Oh, let's don't talk about that, we'll talk about it another time.'"*

Parents can be equally reluctant, however, as described by one adult daughter:

> *"My mother refuses to talk about these things. She assumes I know what she wants ... It's just like, she doesn't want to see the end result. I'd like to discuss what she would like, but she will not discuss it ... She puts an end to the subject."*

Some Non-planners were able to identify circumstances that would cue them to begin thinking about a long-term care plan.

"I think you probably start thinking about it when your health is changing, not even necessarily a crisis, just the realization that you are getting pretty old ... that time is fleeting. I don't feel we're there yet.

If you're in fairly good health you don't think about it. You adjust your life ... as things come up. When the time comes that one is incapacitated, then you'll do something. I guess I don't look too far ahead."

What triggers a sense in Pre-planners or Planners, even Risk Choosers, that the risk of dependency merits attention now? In contrast to those who were discouraged from thinking about planning, others were provoked or pressured by family or friends to regard thinking about long-term care as timely. As one Planner's friend said, *"Do it now!"*

Several Planners or Pre-planners mentioned the value of planning now, while they "still had [their] sanity." Some are motivated to think about planning now by current conditions they understand may become worse, requiring long-term care. For these people, fears of financial devastation and dependency on Medicaid are compelling. This may create a sense of timeliness, if not urgency.

Some Planners had witnessed examples of the value of planning now and/or of the consequences of waiting until it was "too late."

"We have seen what other couples have together, moving in [to a CCRC] before that point when they are on their last legs, and that is really very inspirational ... ".

For one participant, a Planner who had self-insured for a long-term care contingency, planning "started fifty years ago."

"My earliest understanding about money came during the worst of the Depression. Every time I had a dime in my pocket, my first thought was, put it away, you may need it, and I've lived that premise. So, I've always tried to provide ahead for what I would need at a later date."

Perception of Responsibility: *Whose responsibility is this?*

Having met the conditions of perceived vulnerability and timeliness, an individual will continue to move toward the Pre-planning phase only if he or she feels, at least in part, ownership of responsibility for care and related planning.

The two major providers of long-term care for disabled older adults are family and government, with family providing the overwhelming proportion of care. Next we discuss these two forms of long-term care.

Family Responsibility

When individuals believe that the responsibility for their care rests with family, they are unlikely to take personal responsibility for developing a plan. One Non-planner delegated responsibility to his family, acquiescing to the major decision of nursing home placement:

> *"I didn't request [being here]. I turned everything over to my kid and it's in his hands. They are in charge of everything for the simple reason I thought they were the proper ones to do it."*

Another Non-planner expressed strong sentiments that long-term care is a family responsibility and that she believed she could rely on it.

> *"I think children should take care of their parents and that the parents should feel welcome. I just think it's something that should be done if at all possible. I think I would be welcome [in my son's home]. I don't think it'd be a problem."*

With few exceptions, however, Non-planners, Pre-planners, Planners, and Risk Choosers alike fervently expressed a wish not to burden their children with responsibility for their care.

> *"The lifestyles of adult children now are so busy that they can't do it anymore, they are scattered all over and a lot of them are working, and they have their own problems, and I would never want to do that to them."*

One participant described a "real covenant" in her family that parents not burden their children.

> *"In our family ... it's very historical; every generation ... we ... say that we will never live with our children."*

Although most participants in this study vehemently expressed a belief that long-term care should not be the burden of adult children, many of the adult child participants argued that an expectation of care came from them. The adult children shared a perception of filial responsibility for assuming at least some of the burden for long-term care. The range of this perceived burden is variable, however. One adult daughter described her role as a listener.

> *"My role with my mother was to listen to her decide [about moving to a CCRC], and it took her five years to decide. This mother asked little more*

of her daughter. It wasn't as though I could be helpful with the decision. She really didn't want me to help her to decide . . . she just wanted me to listen."

At the other end of the responsibility continuum, one daughter described her assumption of full responsibility for her mother's welfare.

"Finally I said, You're coming home with me. She didn't put up a fight."

At least one participant expressed that children could not be relied on to be responsible for long-term care.

"Your kids may be tremendous today, but you don't know what they're going to be like two days from now."

Some participants had no family and others had no reliable family. This reduced the possibilities for assumption of burden to self and government. It was evident that these people felt personally responsible at least by default.

"I have no one to look after me. I have no people. My people are all gone. I don't depend on nobody but myself."

Government Responsibility

Few participants alluded to the responsibility of government to provide care through Medicaid or other public support. Those individuals who did regarded such support as having been earned through a personal history of hard work and tax paying. One nursing home resident remarked:

"I am on Medicare or Medicaid or something. I worked all the time to get it. I've worked ever since I was big enough to work."

Another Non-planner expressed a belief that Medicaid would provide for her and her husband's care. Her attitude toward Medicaid, and toward nursing homes, was clearly less negative than that of most participants. In response to a question about how she anticipated long-term care would be paid for, she responded:

"Medicaid. I mean, when your money's gone it's gone and you're on Medicaid . . . I think you can get fairly good care in the right nursing home on Medicaid, the same custodial care that you would if you were paying for it."

In contrast, a Planner lamented the effect of recent social policies on the erosion of personal and family responsibility for long-term care:

"Over the period of the last twenty years, something happened in the family that now there is [the idea] that the state is supposed to handle this problem.... [I]n the age past, you kept those resources within the family so that you could cover for yourself."

For the most part, participants expressed a perception of shared responsibility. Although they assumed responsibility for their own care, they anticipated some support from family and their fair share of earned support from government.

Perception of Control: *Who has control?*

Even when individuals have a value of personal responsibility for their own welfare, they may feel powerless to influence their own circumstances and make their own choices. According to locus of control theory, individuals with an internal locus of control perceive events to be controllable by themselves; those with an external locus of control perceive events to be in the hands of fate or in the control of powerful others, such as family members, doctors, and so forth (Levenson, 1974; Rotter, 1966). The latter are unlikely to plan for an event that they see as being in someone else's hands. Those with an internal locus of control feel empowered to gather information and participate in other pre-planning activities that will facilitate their personal objectives. They have a sense of power to shape the plan.

The nursing home residents demonstrated the most striking examples of external locus of control among the other focus group participants. This clearly contributed to their status as Non-planners. Most of these participants clearly indicated the powerful force of family or professionals in their long-term care decisions, particularly at a time of crisis. It is perhaps the crises that rendered these individuals "powerless," at least in their perceptions of themselves in their situations.

"My son ... had me to come here. There wasn't much talk."

For some Non-planners loss of control is expected along with dependency.

"Any choices or decisions I have to make for myself. That's the way I want it. Of course, if I get so that I can't make decisions, then they'll have to do the best they can."

Adult children participants provided helpful insights into their role in these issues of control. Their involvement in their parents' long-term care decisions illustrates the potential for ambiguity and confusion. Whose decision is this? Whose objectives are these? Three participants had parents living in CCRCs, and had been relatively passive in any discussions while the CCRC decision was made. These children appeared especially deferential to their parents' wishes and decisions and expressed full support of them. In other cases, however, the reluctance to discuss issues and/or the confusion of responsibility with regard to control appeared to impede progress toward long-term care planning. Clearly linked to issues of filial responsibility are issues of control. Adult children who take some of the responsibility for their parents' care may become "powerful others" in their parents' perception of control. And, adult children with the best of intentions may reluctantly assume or readily embrace control. In most cases, the children assume control when the parents are perceived as dependent on others for care or in making decisions about care. A shift in control is most likely to occur in the midst or aftermath of a crisis.

> *"It was our decision because of her despondency. She was losing weight and talking about wanting to die. [If I had not intervened] she would not have received any of the services."*

The adult children's assumption of control is reflected in the language "let her" go home, "made him" come home, "took her" to day care, "got him" to go, "I started" the services, "I got" some services, and so forth. It is defended in many cases by the belief that the parent's decision-making capacity is impaired.

> *"When it comes to judgment ... she wouldn't have the slightest idea what she was even looking at! I mean, I think I always feel like as our parents get older, we become the parents and they become the children. I mean, when they really get up in years, they really become dependent on our input."*

One daughter described the manner in which she and her sister guide their mother's decisions.

> *"We sort of lead her in a certain direction but we let her think she is still in the lead."*

While allowing her mother the illusion of control, this daughter was still able to achieve a particular outcome that was compatible with her mother's goals.

In contrast, many Pre-planners and Planners were working to preserve future autonomy by struggling for control now. Many participants articulated a need for control and emphasized how much effort they exercised in order to maintain it.

"I don't want someone else to have to do this for me if I can do it for myself."

One participant asserted that, although loss of control may occur someday, it is important to delegate future, substituted control for that eventuality. This she described as a planning behavior.

"I think you need to talk with one of your children; or with your child, so that they know what's going on, and maybe have a Power of Attorney so that when the time comes they can carry right on ... "

PRE-PLANNING PHASE

Years of thinking, in the form of wondering, imagining, and musing about issues of vulnerability, responsibility, and control, may pass before a person enters the Pre-planning phase and takes an inventory of personal resources. Information gathered in this phase is added to, or used to modify, knowledge already accumulated through everyday sources and experiences. Obviously, not all participants had reached the Pre-planning phase; however, all participants possessed some level of information about long-term care, whether or not they had engaged in the active pursuit of it. Therefore, even those who had not met the first condition of Perception of Vulnerability, or those for whom thinking about long-term care was not timely, or those for whom decisions were perceived to be out of their control, had *some* information, however adequate or accurate, about long-term care. Therefore, even Non-planners contributed to our understanding of the quality and level of information found among the 43 participants.

Adequacy of Information: *Do I have the needed information?*

For informed planning decisions, individuals need adequate knowledge of policies, programs, options (including local services), costs, and eligibility requirements. In addition, being armed with information about the course and prognosis of their existing illnesses or conditions enables individuals to better anticipate future needs. Participants in this study who were in the Pre-planning phase or beyond shared numerous accounts of information-seeking activities.

Accuracy of Information

Although many participants were armed with accurate information about such things as nursing home costs and the limits of Medicaid, some participants appeared to fill information gaps with assumptions that were sometimes accurate, sometimes erroneous.

> *"I think Social Security pays the whole thing (nursing home care). Some information was infused with rumor."*

In the following case, the rumored shortcomings of in-home care led to the conclusion that it was an undesirable option.

> *"You could live in your place and have help come in and help you. But they don't always show up. They don't wanna come at night. They don't want to work holidays or Saturdays or Sundays."*

Long-term care insurance has only recently achieved a relatively high profile in the popular media and among participants there was wide variability in their related knowledge. Many participants demonstrated limited understanding about long-term care insurance and readily admitted the insufficiency of their knowledge in this area. Some were overwhelmed by the "small print" and uncertain about costs and criteria for participation.

Sources of Information

Several participants, both Planners and Non-planners, revealed a lack of information through their questions or through statements to others in the group. Some participants acknowledged this absence of information; others, however, were unaware of the existence of the information at all. In one Non-planner's words, information was received,

> *"Catch as catch can ... We're not aware of what's available. No one explained it to us. No one offered information pertaining to it."*

Several Pre-planners described the sometimes frustrating experience of information seeking, portraying themselves as floundering, without direction or guidance. Until they made their CareChoice Ohio contact, there was no clear sense among these participants that a source of information was available to them.

"I did not know [of] these [long-term care] organizations. I had never heard of them. Because I had been fishing, fishing, fishing ... nobody knew anything ... you know, about these things."

Adult children, assuming responsibility and control for their parents' welfare, were frequently engaged in information seeking and gathering, mostly in response to an immediate need. Their long-term care-related activities suggested a system of crisis management, with only minimal crisis anticipation and prevention. Therefore, the adult children were seldom instruments of the development of a long-term care plan but were important sources of information and linkages to services.

The Planners appeared to have had particular success or fortune in information gathering. For some, this was serendipitous, for others, deliberate.

"There was quite a layout in the newspaper, where they listed all the different insurance companies and all the goods and bads. It was quite a super list of options."

One Pre-planner credited her living in an urban area with enhancing her access to information, and another aggressively pursued information through the mail:

"I live in Columbus and I consider myself very fortunate ... that they put out a lot of literature quickly on what's new. And I read as much as possible to keep current."

"I sent to AARP. They have very good information and ... the Department of Aging puts out a book they call the Senior Handbook, but they list all kinds of resources."

Trustworthiness of Information

Even when information is understood, it may not be trusted. Several participants expressed concern about being able to trust the sources of information available to them. For many, conflicting messages rendered all information untrustworthy and an impediment to planning, as suggested by this Pre-planner:

"Another thing is all this information you get through the mail from insurances and you wonder, can you trust the company? And you see the advertisements on TV, these older actors saying well they rely on it ... but how can you be sure?"

Finally, one participant, a Non-planner, suggested that information is adequate only as long as it is current, and that what we understand about policies and programs today may be irrelevant tomorrow, given the changing tide of sentiment toward public entitlements and private responsibility. She summed it up simply:

> *"How sure are we of Medicaid?" Another group member replied, "We can't be confident of anything."*

Costs and Eligibility

Very much on the minds of most participants was the financial cost of long-term care. For some participants, it appeared that a perception of the high costs of care inhibited their sense of control, thereby discouraging further thinking toward planning. With descriptors such as "prohibitive" or "ridiculous," they abandoned any notion that meeting these costs was within the realm of possibility. Those who maintained a sense of control and sought further information used information about costs to assess the adequacy of their personal resources and the viability of a plan.

As stated earlier, many participants were informed about the costs of nursing home care. Few provided information to the researchers, accurate or otherwise, about the costs of in-home care. General observations about long-term care costs were the rule:

> *"Now, you either have to have nothing or have a potful, a bottomless pit. The middle class, where we are, falls through the cracks and has to pay. If you don't have anything, you go on Medicaid and of course if you are a Rockefeller ... you can have nurses around the clock to take care of you."*

Although general observations contribute to information, only individuals who were adequately and accurately informed about policies, programs, costs, and requirements moved successfully to, and engage effectively in, the next requirement on the planning path: Perception of Resources.

Perception of Resources: *Do I have the needed resources?*

Financial Resources

With the exception of the Planners, the vast majority of participants perceived themselves to have insufficient resources to afford long-term care planning. Claiming fixed or limited incomes, limited savings, or the financial devastation of medical expenses already incurred, these individuals described the costs of long-term care planning, particularly of long-term care insurance, as "too expensive," "prohibitive," "ridiculous," "too high," "an arm and a leg," and "out of reach."

It is clear that many participants were caught off guard by the perceived mismatch between projected long-term care costs and their capacities to afford them. They expressed a combination of dismay and hopelessness.

> *"Everybody here put money aside for their own upkeep later on. We thought we were doing it. I've lost a lot of hope."*

It is evident that many individuals, relying on a superficial assessment of their financial status, do not take a thorough personal inventory of financial capacity to plan for long-term care costs. For those who do, some find that it comes too late, that indeed, although they might have once had sufficient resources to accumulate toward this need over time, the cost is now prohibitive. Finally, some individuals have never had discretionary resources to commit to a long-term care plan. A perception of limited financial resources can lead to a sense of futility and a failure to take stock of personal, non-financial assets and supports. As one Non-planner said:

> *"I don't know what you* **can** *plan. What* **can** *you plan if you don't have long-term care insurance?"*

Social/Environmental Resources

What happens to individuals armed with adequate information but without sufficient resources to make a rational decision to commit to a long-term care financial plan? Though their planning options are limited, these individuals may develop other strategies for preparing for the possibility of long-term care dependency.

A social/environmental plan may be characterized by a number of decisions, all of which were represented among the study participants. Individuals who change or adapt housing to prepare for the possibility of future limitations in mobility enhance the likelihood of living independently for a longer period of time. Those individuals who move to be nearer to informal social supports, particularly family, expand their base of potential caregiver support. One Pre-planner without family sought to share her home with someone, having decided that it

> *"Isn't really safe for someone [my] age to be living alone."*

This woman regarded her home as an asset she could exchange for care.

"Well, there are lots of people who need a place to live and I have that."

A social/environmental plan may also include informing oneself about the range of long-term care service options, and making preferences about these options clear to one's social support network, so that in the event of a crisis, decisions about services may be made more expeditiously and appropriately.

"I don't know what I'm gonna need in the future, but I want to know what's available to me to make good decisions."

Finally, a social/environmental long-term care plan may include legal arrangements and agreements with family or other designated individuals who can make health care decisions consistent with the wishes of the older adult. Several participants in this study had designated a Durable Power of Attorney for Health Care, and several had signed living wills.

The reality of a social/environmental plan is that, without a way to afford a full range of care options over an extended period of time, there cannot exist full protection against the consequences of long-term care dependency. Housing changes, living arrangements, and legal agreements can only go so far to enhance options and reduce the public burden of Medicaid expenditures.

Combined Resources for Comprehensive Planning

Optimal preparation for long-term care contingencies includes a combination of financial planning, adaptations in housing or living arrangements, the development and maintenance of a social support system, education about services, and legal agreements for health care and other decisions. The members of the Insured group had not only committed financial resources toward long-term care but *also* engaged in most other forms of planning.

RATIONAL DECISION

Even when an individual determines that he or she has sufficient financial, social, or environmental resources to invest in a long-term care plan, a rational decision must be made to invest time, energy, and resources now toward an unpredictable future. Although long-term-care planning requires a perception of vulnerability, long-term care dependency is often perceived as a possibility—at most, a probability—but is rarely perceived as a certainty. Except in the cases of preexisting degenerative conditions such as Alzheimer's disease, the likelihood of long-term care dependency is essentially unknowable and unpredictable. Healthy, independent individuals considering an investment toward an uncertain future must weigh their perceived risk against the costs of the investment.

Deciding to Commit to a Plan: *Do I choose to invest time, energy, and/or resources now toward an unpredictable future?*

Many Planners regarded their decisions to commit to a financial plan as a means of protecting both their children (from the burden of care) and their assets (from depletion).

> *"I had annuities put away back a long time ago to pay all expenses so that I didn't need to worry about it. For the good of the family, . . . and who knows what their futures hold. . . . "*

Choosing Risk

Like the Planners, Risk Choosers had moved through the six earlier stages of the planning path and had achieved a point of rational decision. Unlike the Planners, however, Risk Choosers decided not to commit resources toward the risk of long-term care dependency, but to forego planning and take their chances.

> *"I've read the literature and I decided I didn't want to get involved with that: spending all the money to do that. It would be easier . . . I mean I could end up . . . it's a gamble. I could end up where I really need it, or I could spend thousands and die of a heart attack or something."*

The decision to "gamble" rather than to plan may be the result of an informed, deliberate process. Without a catalyst that would alter their weighing of the costs and benefits of making a plan, Risk Choosers are unlikely to commit time and resources toward a comprehensive long-term care plan.

REVIEW AND REVISION

As stated earlier, effective planning requires continual review and revision according to changes in perceptions, needs, options, and resources.

One Planner described switching from one insurance company to another, whereas another described in detail the attention he keeps on his finances and related communications (updates) with his daughter. Another Planner had bought long-term care insurance and was looking toward a move to a CCRC in another 5 years.

CONCLUSION

Each of the seven conditions necessary to arrive at a plan for long-term care represents significant challenges to the average individual. Acknowledging and accepting one's own vulnerability to a period of dependency in late life is a difficult achievement. Without a recognition of personal vulnerability, however, the inertia of "doing nothing" cannot be overcome. It is clear that there is no magic trigger to provoke people into a perception of vulnerability. The triggers varied in intensity and type among the participants in this study.

A perception of timeliness appears almost as challenging. What drives a 66-year-old to purchase long-term-care insurance, whereas a 68-year-old argues that it is "not time" to think about such matters. What brings an 84-year-old to decide it is now time to "plan ahead"? There does not appear to be a magic moment or age at which individuals arrive at a sense of timeliness. Again, triggers varied in intensity and type.

There is considerable variation in ideas about personal, family, and government responsibility for long-term care. The mixed messages sent by both family members and government serve to confuse, if not erode, perceptions of personal responsibility for care. For at least one participant, the availability of Medicaid support for nursing home care was regarded, if not as a plan, at least as a safety net.

Personal control in long-term care decision making appears to be at risk in the more vulnerable individuals, characteristic of the nursing home residents and the adult children's parents, many of whom were receiving some type of long-term care services. Few of these individuals appeared to be at the center of control of their futures, and it was not surprising that they had become passive about long-term care decisions and plans. Also threatened by loss of personal control were individuals who believed that their precarious financial circumstances put plans about their care at the mercy of others.

Participants in this study shared a wide array of experiences and attitudes about information sources and information gathering. They expressed concerns about identifying appropriate sources for information and were especially concerned about the accuracy and trustworthiness of information they had received. Several participants acknowledged ignorance about policies, programs, costs, and eligibility, whereas others expressed confidence that they were sufficiently informed. Nearly all expressed an understanding that policies and programs change and that this flux requires vigilance on the part of the consumer.

Among participants, a wide variation in the perception of resources for long-term care reflected a wide range of socioeconomic backgrounds. Even so, the more "privileged" of the participants appeared quick to decide that they had inadequate resources. With the exception of the Planners, few seemed to have taken the thorough personal inventory necessary for a rational decision. Regarding informal social supports as a resource, few participants had discussions with their children to clarify expectations about caregiving.

The knowledge gained from this focus group study about the path to long-term care planning offers a foundation for understanding how to encourage and facilitate planning and provide appropriate information to individuals at all stages of the long-term care planning process. Individual and family choices about long-term care are clearly enhanced through planning, with faces toward the future. Policies, programs, and practices that promote long-term care planning must do so with a serious appreciation of its complexity.

ACKNOWLEDGMENTS

An earlier version of this chapter exists in McGrew, K.B., & Straker, J.K. (1996) *Facilitating individual long-term care planning: The role of CareChoice Ohio.* Oxford, OH: Scripps Gerontology Center, Miami University.

This research was funded by the Ohio Department of Aging.

REFERENCES

Cutler, N. E. (1996). Retirement planning and the cost of long-term care: Battling the fear of the unknown. *Journal of the American Society of CLU and ChFC, 50*(6) 42–48.

Foster, L., Brown, R., Phillips, B., Schore, J., & Carlson, B. L. (2003, March). *Improving the quality of Medicaid personal assistance through consumer direction.* Health Affairs, Supplemental Web Exclusives: W3-162–175.

George, L. K. (1993). Sociological Perspectives on Life Transitions. *Annual Review of Sociology 19*: 353–373.

Greenwald, M., & Associates (1999). The NCOA/John Hancock Long-Term Care Survey Executive Summary. Washington, DC: National Council on the Aging and John Hancock.

Harvard School of Public Health and Louis Harris & Associates. (1996). *Long Term Care Awareness Survey*, January 6.

Kaiser Family Foundation. (2001, October). *National survey of nursing homes.* Menlo Park, CA: Author.

Levenson, H. (1974). Activism and powerful others: Distinctions with the concept of internal-external control. *Journal of Personality Assessment, 38*(4), 7738.

McGrew, K. B., & Straker, J. K. (1996). *Facilitating individual long-term care planning: The role of CareChoice Ohio.* Oxford, OH: Scripps Gerontology Center, Miami University.

Mebane, F. (2001). Want to understand how Americans viewed long-term care in 1998? Start with media coverage. *The Gerontologist, 41*(1), 24.

Rotter, J. B. (1966). Generalized expectancies for internal versus external control of reinforcement. *Psychological Monographs, 80*(1),1–28.

San Antonio, P. M., & Rubenstein, R. L. (2004). Long-term care planning as a cultural system. *Journal of Aging & Social Policy, 16*(2), 35–48.

Sörensen, S., & Pinquart, M. (2000). Preparation for future care needs: Styles of preparation used by older Eastern German, United States, and Canadian women. *Journal of Cross-Cultural Gerontology, 15*(4), 349–381.

Sörensen, S., & Zarit, S. H. (1996). Preparation for caregiving: A study of multi-generation families. *International Journal of Aging & Human Development, 42*(1), 43–63.

Strauss, A. (1987). *Qualitative analysis for social scientists.* Cambridge: Cambridge University Press.

PART II

Consumer Voice

CHAPTER EIGHT

Capturing the Voices of Consumers in Long-Term Care:

If You Ask Them They Will Tell

Robert A. Applebaum
Gwen C. Uman
Jane K. Straker

The magazine *Consumer Reports* has become a mainstay of American society, reaching 4.5 million subscribers with their print version and another 325,000 who subscribe to reports online (answers.com, 2005). Whether considering an automobile purchase, exploring the new flat-screen, high-definition, plasma television set, or hearing about customer service at hotels across America, consumers want to know about the experiences of others. Society has developed extensive consumer satisfaction and feedback mechanisms to assess how we feel about the appliances we buy, our auto-repair experience, and to ascertain how we were treated at the local fast-food restaurant. Industries from airlines to zoos have long used consumer input to improve their services, increase their market share, and as they hope, to increase their profits.

One growing and important industry that has only recently received the attention of consumers is long-term care. In 2004, private long-term care expenditures for nursing homes, assisted living facilities, and in-home services topped the $100 billion mark. Also in 2004, public expenditures through Medicaid, Medicare, and other state-funded programs accounted for an additional $100 billion (Burwell, 2004; Congressional Budget Office [CBO], 2004). Clearly long-term care is a major U.S. industry. Yet until recently, only limited efforts have been made to ask how those who receive long-term care fare. Such a belated recognition of the importance of consumer satisfaction is in many ways surprising given the personal nature of long-term care. Of all consumer services, what could be more important than how one is treated by the person who helps with the most private tasks of daily living, such as bathing, dressing, and toileting?

It was not until 2000 that *Consumer Reports* published their first nursing home "watch list"—a listing of facilities with chronic poor performance on their annual Medicare and Medicaid certification surveys. Several privately operated web sites (MyZiva.net, Healthgrades.com) provide similar survey-based information about nursing homes. A number of states and the federal Centers for Medicare and Medicaid Services (CMS) now have some form of quality assessment information on the Internet (e.g., consumer guides), although only a small minority includes the perspectives of long-term care consumers—residents and families (Castle & Lowe, 2005).

There are several reasons why getting input from consumers about long-term care services has been limited in the past. First, it is more difficult to survey this group of consumers than purchasers of other products and services. Furthermore, consumers who require long-term assistance often have health conditions, sensory impairments, or cognitive limitations that make surveys more difficult to complete. In many instances consumers may have cognitive diseases, such as Alzheimer's or other forms of dementia, that can limit their ability to respond to questions asked by phone, mail, or even in person. Second, consumers participating in publicly funded programs, in some cases, may be fearful that negative responses to questions about their services could adversely affect the care they receive. Often when providers have collected information from consumers, it has not been made clear how such data are to be used, causing consumers to question their involvement in such an exercise (Applebaum, Straker, & Geron, 2000; Coleman, 2000). Finally, both professionals and family members tend to hold negative attitudes in regard to the ability of older consumers to assess and advocate for their own care needs. A major barrier to using information from consumers in long-term care has been an assumption that older people with chronic physical and cognitive disabilities simply cannot provide valid and reliable opinions about their services.

In recent years there has been increasing success on the part of the long-term care research community in developing and testing surveys that long-term care consumers can reliably respond to. Evidence suggests that some of the negative regulator, provider, and family attitudes are changing (Applebaum et al., 2000; Geron, Smith, Tennstedt, Jette, Chassler, &

Kasten, 2000; Kane et al., 2003; Uman & Urman, 1998). As previously mentioned several states have included resident satisfaction findings in their consumer guides (Castle & Lowe, 2005) and at least one state (MN) incorporates resident satisfaction as a factor in their reimbursement formula. The Eighth Scope of Work for Quality Improvement Organizations (QIOs) in each state calls for annual resident and staff satisfaction surveys. (QIOs are organizations in each state that contract with CMS to oversee quality improvement activities for hospitals, nursing homes, home care agencies, and other Medicare providers.)

Our experience in assessing the satisfaction of consumers using long-term care is that in the majority of cases, consumers can indeed provide meaningful feedback about the services or assistance they receive. This feedback typically captures the perceptions of consumers and has proven to be useful in quality management activities.

In this chapter, we draw on experiences with three projects designed to gain input from consumers in the in-home and nursing home settings.

1. A series of projects undertaken by Vital Research, LLC (VR), a private research firm, to develop a nursing home Resident Satisfaction Interview (RSI) part of the Resident Experience and Assessment of Life (REAL) system.
2. Work by the Scripps Gerontology Center to create a satisfaction survey for Ohio nursing home residents (Ohio Nursing Home Resident Satisfaction Survey, or ONHRSS) and family members (Ohio Nursing Home Family Satisfaction Survey).
3. Work by researchers at Scripps, in conjunction with the Ohio Department of Aging (ODA) and the Council on Aging of Southwestern Ohio to modify the Home Care Satisfaction Measure (HCSM) designed by Geron and his colleagues. Designed for administration by care managers, the new instrument is known as the Service Adequacy and Satisfaction Instrument (SASI).

Our discussion about these efforts will focus on three areas of importance: (1) instrument development, (2) processes and methods of data collection, and (3) analysis and use of data for quality improvement.

The instruments discussed are part of an array of tools now being developed to assess consumer satisfaction (Applebaum et al., 2000; Cohen-Mansfield, Ejaz, & Werner, 2000). They are presented first as examples of the approaches used and then to demonstrate the fact that with careful instrument development and rigorous data-collection methods consumers can assess and communicate their feelings about the quality of services received. The best choice of an instrument for a particular program depends on a range of factors such as the type of program, type of consumer, what resources are available for data collection, and how the program administrators intends to use the results. The most important message of this chapter is not that there is one best way to collect consumer satisfaction data; rather, it is that in the majority of instances consumers who receive long-term supports can assess and communicate their views on service satisfaction.

INSTRUMENT DEVELOPMENT

The techniques used for developing these instruments have common elements. These instruments were developed using a consumer-focused qualitative process, followed by a quantitative pilot test, and final refinement prior to full-scale implementation.

Qualitative Process

The qualitative process was undertaken to identify the areas that were most relevant to consumers regarding their satisfaction with long-term care services. Two techniques have been used to develop instruments of this type: individual interviews and focus groups. To develop the RSI (Uman, 1996; Uman & Urman, 1997) investigators divided a sample of nursing home residents into groups based on cognitive ability, using the Cognitive Performance Scale (Hartmaier, Sloane, Guess, & Koch, 1994). Thirty interviews were conducted with individuals representing a range of cognitive abilities in two nursing homes; one nursing home had a high proportion of African-American residents. In-person interviews using semistructured and open-ended questions were used to ask residents about what they liked and disliked about living in the facility. Interview responses were then content analyzed, and six consumer requirements or domains of satisfaction were identified including: help and assistance, communication with staff, autonomy and choice, companionship, food and environment, and safety and security. Based on these domains closed ended questions were developed.

The home care survey development process began with the focus group approach, which was then supplemented with in-depth personal interviews. The initial HCSM, developed by Geron and his colleagues (2000), used a series of focus groups with a diverse set of older consumers to establish the areas of importance. Based on these focus groups a closed ended survey was developed and tested. The HCSM, which includes measures in four component areas including consumer–worker relationships, worker competence, worker performance, and agency performance, has been used widely and has been shown to be valid and reliable in its assessment of home care satisfaction (Geron et al., 2000).

The tool described in this chapter, although based on the HCSM, is used in a different way than the original instrument. The HCSM, as developed and as currently implemented, uses research interviewers for data collection. In the work reported in this chapter we wanted to use care managers from each agency administering Ohio's PASSPORT program (the state's Medicaid home- and community-based waiver program) to collect satisfaction data as part of their regularly scheduled in-home visits. Our motivation for this approach was an interest in generating consumer satisfaction data to assess the performance of individual home care providers, rather than simply to examine data at the administrative agency level. To accomplish such a goal, very large sample sizes are needed, and using research interviewers would be prohibitively expensive for agencies. The major advantage of the care manager approach is that care managers can complete the interview as part of their regularly scheduled visit, thus reducing survey costs dramatically. The disadvantage of such an approach is that care managers are not neutral interviewers; they have relationships with their clients as well as the service providers with whom they arrange and monitor services. A separate study in which we compared data collected by research interviewers and care managers found that with proper training care managers could collect data in comparable fashion (Murdoch, Kunkel, Applebaum, & Straker, 2004).

The care managers involved in the testing of this data collection strategy liked the HCSM instrument but expressed an interest in tailoring the tool specifically to their in-home program. For example, the PASSPORT program had adopted a philosophy that gave clients an expectation that in-home workers should be professional and that the worker–consumer relationship should be friendly, but not a close friendship. In developing the original HCSM, focus group members talked about the importance of the worker being a friend to the consumer, and so an item was included about the worker as friend. Care managers, however, felt that such an item should not be included in the instrument administered by their agencies.

To determine the extent and type of changes that care managers thought were necessary, three focus groups were held with care managers. Two of the groups had previously administered the HCSM; the third had not administered the HCSM but responded to survey items based on their experiences with clients and program philosophies. The focus group participants recommended a series of changes to the survey that customized the instrument for their specific program. Based on their suggestions, revisions to the instrument were made that included rewording, deleting and adding some items, and changing response categories.

Item Construction

The developers of both the nursing home and the home care tools attempted to include items representing observable behaviors based on the qualitative data gathered from focus groups and interviews. Traditionally, service quality measures have relied on opinions and attitudes that are personal and based on individually defined criteria. An excellent rating on "courtesy" means many different things to different consumers. In response, instrument design has focused on developing items that ask specific questions. For example, on the RSI, questions were asked, such as Do the people who work here handle you gently? Do the people who work here listen to what you say? On the home care side, items include: my worker works all her hours and my worker follows my instructions. The ONHRSS and SASI use multiple Likert response categories, whereas with the RSI, residents are prompted to give dichotomous "yes" or "no" responses.

Pilot Testing

After items were developed these projects used an extensive pilot-test procedure. The RSI was pilot tested with 300 individuals that included Caucasian and African-American nursing home residents. In this case, the pilot test was used to help finalize the survey, so various response formats (three, four, or five response categories or dichotomous categories) were tested.

As part of the pilot-test subsamples of consumers underwent 1-day or 1-week test–retest procedures to determine the reliability of the satisfaction instrument. Findings from this analysis found that in about 80% of the cases the responses were stable across the two interviews. Interestingly, even in cases where residents had higher levels of cognitive impairment, the instrument was quite stable, and results for this group did not vary widely from the overall sample.

The ONHRSS development used the additional strategy of behavior coding to refine items as part of the pilot test as well as test–retest and interrater reliability interviews with subsamples of residents. For the behavioral coding, a small sample of interviews was videotaped, and the tapes were analyzed for interviewer errors in question reading, respondent requests for repeating the items, requests for clarification, and inability to choose a response. Behavioral coding identified a number of small refinements that were made to improve the structure of items for ease of interviewer reading, and wording modifications were made to improve comprehension for residents.

The ONHRSS also tested a branching strategy that allowed residents who answered a simple "yes" or "no" to be asked whether they meant "yes, always" or "yes, sometimes" instead of reading all four response categories (always, sometimes, hardly ever, and never) when residents initially did not choose an answer. This strategy eliminates some of the complexity in choosing an answer for those with cognitive impairments.

To supplement the pilot test done for SASI, researchers also completed cognitive interviews, in which respondents were asked questions about the survey items after they had completed the initial questionnaire. Twelve cognitive interviews examining item wording and response categories were conducted, and suggestions for additional questions were requested. Respondents were asked to explain the meaning of the questions, and their preferences for wording and response categories. Consumer suggestions were used to make modifications to the instrument, although consumers did not recommend additional items. The revised instrument was then pilot tested by care managers. Care manager interviewers were then debriefed in an effort to identify whether any additional changes were needed. A final step in the instrument development process included another focus group with care managers who had used the original instrument to review the revised tool. Based on their input the instrument was finalized and ready for an extensive pilot test. Interview training materials, including a computer-based video, were developed to prepare care managers to conduct the interviews.

The home care tool was then pretested with 464 clients in two regions of the state. All clients were asked to participate during the regular 6-month assessment visit by the care manager. Clients who were completely noncommunicative or unavailable were the only individuals initially excluded from participating in the survey process. For other interviews, if the client could not choose three appropriate answers in a row the interview was terminated. If a client could not be interviewed, a proxy was used. This process allowed for inclusion of clients with varying levels of impairment. Care managers were strongly encouraged not to make decisions about which clients would be capable of participating in the interviews prior to their visit.

PROCESSES AND METHODS OF DATA COLLECTION

Although costly, our experiences have shown that the preferred strategy for collecting satisfaction information from those receiving long-term care services is in a face-to-face interview. Although written surveys can be used with this population, our desire to include input from as many consumers as possible precludes this strategy. By their nature, written surveys exclude those who have vision, writing, and literacy problems, as well as some of those who have cognitive impairments who can respond to verbal questions.

Our experiences in both the in-home and nursing home settings support the contention that the majority of consumers who receive long-term assistance are able to participate in satisfaction surveys when they are administered in an interview setting. For example, in the more than 14,000 resident interviews that have now been completed by VR using the RSI, more than three-fourths of the residents were able to complete the satisfaction survey. Nine percent of residents refused to participate, and 12% failed the behavioral screening questions used to assess the resident's ability to answer yes or no questions. There is variation in the proportion of residents who are willing and able to respond based on the extent of their cognitive impairment. For example, more than 90% of residents with minimal impairment were willing and able to respond, compared to 42% of those residents with severe impairment.

A review of participation results for the home care survey showed that more than 90% of the clients were able to complete the interviews directly. In about 5% of the cases the client had a legally authorized representative who completed the survey. In 4% of the cases a proxy interview was required, even though the client did not have an authorized representative. In less than 1% of the cases, a client either refused to participate (.02) or terminated the interview (.04). Using care managers who are known to consumers appears to increase completion rates.

Field Implementation

VR has gathered data from nursing home residents using the RSI (14,000 interviews in 250 nursing homes nationwide), the ONHRSS (22,000 interviews in 968 nursing homes in Ohio and Rhode Island), and the Consumer Satisfaction and Quality of Life Survey in Minnesota Nursing Homes (14,000 interviews in 399 nursing homes). Although both nursing home and home care surveys report high response rates, our experience suggests that there are three factors that influence both response rates and measurement accuracy: consumer factors, interviewer factors, and instrument factors. Figure 8.1 presents the detailed components of the three areas.

Consumer Factors

Recipients of long-term services and supports experience chronic disability that can affect their ability to participate in consumer satisfaction

Consumer Factors

- Hearing
- Vision
- Memory
- Capacity to understand
- Attention

Interviewer Factors

- Belief in the resident
- Animation of facial expression
- Inflection of voice
- Appropriate use of hearing amplifiers
- Attention-getting techniques

- Redirection
- Clarification
- Use of silence (pausing)
- Adherence to structured Interview
- Environmental manipulation

Instrument Factors

- Question phrasing
- Prompts
- Alternative phrasing
- Length of questions
- Response format

Figure 8.1 Factors Influencing Measurement of Satisfaction.

surveys. Our experience in interviewing residents of nursing homes found hearing impairment to be a major barrier to successful completion of the interview. Problems of cognitive impairment are compounded by hearing loss; in some cases hearing problems are interpreted as cognitive difficulties. To compensate for hearing loss our projects have used three techniques. First, we have had success with relatively inexpensive portable hearing amplifiers that can be purchased at local electronic stores. Second, interviewers also pay close attention to the environment in which they are conducting the survey; making sure that it supports the hearing needs of the consumer. Eliminating outside noises and distractions is important to improving the communication process. Other environmental issues include making sure that consumers have their glasses and being sure that consumers are not facing any glare so they can see the facial expressions of the interviewer. The type and nature of the questions is also an important factor, particularly with individuals who experience cognitive problems. Shorter, one-step questions help consumers with memory loss to better remember and understand the question. Cognitively impaired consumers also have more difficulty with instruments that use multiple-choice response categories; the branching response strategy (e.g., from a "yes" response to a choice between "yes, always" and "yes, sometimes") helps reduce the complexity of multiple responses.

Interviewer Factors

Skilled and well-trained interviewers can have a major impact on success. One factor of critical importance is that the interviewer believes that every consumer has the capability of reporting on his or her daily life experience. Consumer advocacy underlies the successful survey process. When working with consumers who have cognitive difficulties, it is important to believe that with the right tool, in the right setting, every consumer can successfully report. It is also important that the interviewers have skills such as attention-getting techniques, redirecting, clarifying, and repeating all or parts of the question to obtain accurate information. Our experience indicates that interviewers who do not value the input of consumers or who do not believe that consumers can provide good quality feedback will be less successful.

One finding from the administration of both nursing home resident surveys is that structured interviewing is an acquired skill. In the nursing home resident surveys, at least 3 days of training, which includes didactic material, practice, feedback, a knowledge test, and a performance test, are needed to prepare interviewers for the field. Interestingly, professional clinicians from fields such as medicine, social work, nursing, and gerontology have been more difficult to train, because they tend to prejudge the consumer's ability to respond to the survey without following the procedures designed to include as many residents as possible.

Instrument Factors

Because individuals who receive long-term assistance have physical or cognitive challenges, the instrument can affect the quality of data and response rates. Question phrasing, length of questions, and number of response categories all need to be considered carefully. Keeping questions clear and straightforward is critical. The cognitive interviewing and behavioral coding processes discussed earlier are important ways to make sure that consumers respond to the designed intent of the question. The structure of response categories is one that generates debate in the design of satisfaction surveys. Because it is important to capture the true opinions of consumers' answers, it is useful to offer recipients a range of response categories. However, it is easier for consumers with cognitive disability to answer yes or no to a question than it is to rate their opinion on a 5- or 7-point scale. One option to facilitate data collection when using multiple-response categories is to provide the respondent with a list of response categories as a reminder or prompt as they complete the survey. Classical measurement theory would suggest that the more response choices consumers have, within their ability to discriminate the phenomenon under study, the more variation possible (and hence the greater the reliability of the scores). The two NH instruments described in this chapter offer an opportunity to examine measurement theory as it applies to this frail consumer population. Finally, length of the survey is a strategic decision as well. We have tried to keep the interviews to no more than 20 minutes to avoid fatigue and to minimize dropouts.

ANALYSIS AND USE OF DATA
FOR QUALITY IMPROVEMENT

Although it is the case that the majority of consumers do report high rates of satisfaction with the services they receive, survey results reinforce the conclusion that consumers receiving long-term supports can successfully report on their long-term care experience. For example, a detailed look at the results from the Ohio nursing home resident satisfaction survey implemented with more than 18,000 individuals showed a range of outcomes. In areas such as satisfaction with facility personnel, including nurses aides, activity staff, social workers, and administration, more than 90% of respondents ranked their nursing home positively. An environmental assessment, including both the safety of the facility and the ability to personalize the resident's room were also reported as positive aspects of the services provided. There were also select areas where less than 75% of the residents reported being positive about the facility's effort. For example, areas of resident dissatisfaction were found in areas of choice—specifically in regard to the time the resident gets up in the morning, food (both taste and availability), laundry services, and staff interactions.

Results from the home care survey completed with over 4,000 consumers are presented in Table 8.1. Overall, consumers report high rates of service satisfaction. However, in some dimensions of service such as workers keeping to their scheduled times, working all of their assigned hours, and doing things the way the client wants, there was more variation on satisfaction with services. Consumers were able to identify instances where they felt that service quality could be improved.

Table 8.1 Sample Provider Quality Report: A Closer Look

	Always	Usually	Sometimes	Hardly Ever	Never
Workers work all their hours	78%	13%	5%	3%	1%
Workers keep their scheduled hours	68%	27%	3%	1%	1%
Clients can depend on their workers	79%	19%	1%	0%	1%
Workers know how to do their job	82%	14%	3%	0%	1%
Workers do a good job	71%	22%	5%	1%	1%
Workers know what to do	79%	16%	4%	0%	1%
Workers follow clients' instructions	82%	13%	3%	1%	1%
Workers do things the way clients want	73%	21%	5%	0%	1%
Workers care about clients as people	89%	7%	3%	0%	1%
Clients trust their workers	89%	8%	2%	0%	1%
Workers treat client with respect	92%	6%	1%	0%	1%
Clients are told changes in workers' schedule	74%	16%	5%	3%	2%

One important aspect about the collection of consumer satisfaction data is determining how to use it to improve services. All of the surveys discussed in this chapter are currently being used extensively. The ONHRSS results are posted on a consumer website developed by the ODA. The web site (www.ltcohio.org) is designed to provide information to potential residents and their families about nursing homes in the state. The web site includes results from the state survey and other regulatory quality domains, but the core components of the web site are satisfaction data from consumers and their families. Survey results are presented by facility, so that consumers can have better information to assist in making selection decisions. In addition to the survey scores, individuals using the web site are provided with information on how the facility being examined compares to the rest of the state. Although resident and family satisfaction scores are only one piece of information needed for making a selection decision, thousands of consumers call on these data to assist them with the decision-making process each month. A secondary goal of the legislation that established the consumer website was the improvement of nursing home care in Ohio. Evidence suggests that providers use the satisfaction data to help them improve satisfaction with care (Uman, Urman, & Young, 1998). In Rhode Island, nursing homes have also requested assistance with establishing priorities for service improvements based on results from surveys of residents and families.

The home care satisfaction results have been used in a different way than the nursing home data. Rather than communicate findings directly to consumers, the home care results are used by the contracting agency in working with the direct service providers to help to improve the quality of services. In this case, the area agency involved with the study publishes a provider report each quarter that includes satisfaction results. Providers are able to review their results in the context of similar providers. The report also includes a range of scores and the ranking of each provider. The provider is able to compare its score to both a relative comparison of other providers and an absolute benchmark established by the area agency. In some instances, providers request technical assistance from the area agency when scores are below expectations.

Although consumer satisfaction results are used quite differently in the two examples presented, they highlight the importance of consumer input in improving the quality of services. In both examples results form consumers have become core components of efforts designed to improve the quality of services received. Whether or not consumers use these data, our message is that this information is integral to quality assurance and quality improvement efforts.

CONCLUSION

Despite some major barriers faced in efforts to assess the satisfaction of consumers receiving long-term care services and supports, this chapter highlights that most consumers can indeed be successfully involved in this endeavor. Our experience indicates that consumers with physical and cognitive disabilities are able, in the majority of cases, to actively participate in consumer satisfaction efforts. These data can clearly be used to better inform consumers and providers about the services delivered, and as part of a quality management system designed to improve services.

The design and delivery of long-term care services and supports has been consistently criticized for ignoring the consumer. Whether the criticism focuses on the lack of balance in the system, the lack of consumer choice and options, or concerns about quality of services, the fundamental problem is that consumer needs have been largely ignored. Ultimately, our ability to improve the quality of long-term care services and supports will only truly happen when we place the consumer at the heart of the delivery system. Without hearing the consumers' voice this goal cannot be achieved.

REFERENCES

Answers.com. (2005). Retrieved August 8, 2005, from www.answers.com/Consumer%20Reports.

Applebaum, R. A., Straker, J. K., & Geron, S. M. (2000). Assessing satisfaction in health and long-term care. New York: Springer.

Burwell, B. (2004). Medicaid long term care expenditures in FY 2003. MedStat. Unpublished.

Castle, N. G., & Lowe, T. J. (2005). Report cards and nursing homes. *The Gerontologist, 45,* 48–67.

Cohen-Mansfield, J., Ejaz, F. K., & Werner, P. (Eds.). (2000). Satisfaction surveys in long-term care. New York: Springer.

Coleman, B. (2000). Assuring the quality of home care: The challenge of involving the consumer. Issue Brief, AARP. Washington, DC.

Congressional Budget Office. (2004). Financing long-term care for the elderly. Washington, DC.

Geron, S. M., Smith, K., Tennstedt, S., Jette, A., Chassler, D., & Kasten, L. (2000). The home care satisfaction measure: A client-centered approach to assessing the satisfaction of frail older adults with home care services. *Journals of Gerontology Series B: Psychological Sciences & Social Sciences, 55B*(5), S259.

Hartmaier, S. L., Sloane, P. D., Guess, H. A., & Koch, G. G. (1994). The MDS cognition scale: a valid instrument for identifying and staging nursing home residents with dementia using the minimum data set. *Journal of the American Geriatrics Society, 42*(11), 1212.

Kane, R. A., Kling, K. C., Bershadsky, B., Kane, R. L., Giles, K., Degenholtz, H. B., Liu, J., & Cutler, L. J. (2003). Quality of life measures for nursing home residents. *Journals of Gerontology Series B: Psychological Sciences & Social Sciences, 58,* M240.

Murdoch, L. D., Kunkel, S. R., Applebaum, R. A., & Straker, J. K. (2004). Care managers as research interviewers: A test of a strategy for gathering consumer satisfaction. *Journal of Applied Gerontology, 23*(3), 234.

Uman, G. (1996, May). *Quality of life in nursing homes from a consumer research perspective.* Paper presented at the Health Care Financing Administration Symposium: Improving quality of life for nursing home residents; the challenge and the opportunities. Baltimore: Health Care Financing Administration.

Uman, G. C., & Urman, H. N. (1997) Measuring consumer satisfaction in nursing home residents. *Nutrition, 13*(78), 705–707.

Uman, G. C., Urman, H. N., & Young, R. (1998, Winter). Using consumer surveys in long term care today for a better tomorrow. *The Consultant Dietitian, 22*(3), 11–14.

CHAPTER NINE

Caregivers as Consumers:
Perspectives on Quality

Suzanne R. Kunkel
Kathryn B. McGrew
Robert A. Applebaum
Shawn L. Davis

BACKGROUND

Families have historically been the primary provider of long-term care for older Americans. Almost 25 years ago, the General Accounting Office (GAO) estimated that more than 80% of all long-term care was provided by families (GAO, 1977). Since that time, there has been a continued increase in the size of the disabled older population, particularly in the proportion of the oldest old, those who are most likely to need long-term assistance. At the same time, social change such as an increasing number of dual-worker households has altered the family's capacity to provide assistance. The increasingly prevalent role of caregiver requires enormous emotional, physical, and financial efforts, even though it is often willingly undertaken and a source of great personal satisfaction (Kunkel, Applebaum, & Nelson, 2004; Levine, Reinhard, Feinberg, Albert, & Hart, 2004). A recent national survey of older Americans found that more than 7 million caregivers assist more than 4 million disabled older people residing in the community (Administration on Aging [AOA], 2000). Recognizing that families remain the backbone of our long-term care system, the 2000 Older Americans Act established the National Family Caregiver Support Program (NFCSP). Other recent initiatives, including programs

141

that allow family members to be paid for some of the care they are providing and state-funded respite services also speak to the increasing importance of supporting family caregivers.

Caregiver support programs seek to reduce caregiver burden and stress through supportive services and to improve the quality of care the family provides (Greene & Feinberg, 1999). Despite these important goals and the growth in caregiver support services there has been little work examining the quality of services designed to assist family caregivers (Kane & Penrod, 1995; Institute of Medicine [IOM], 2001). Even more problematic, efforts to ask caregivers directly about how they view the quality of services have been quite limited. Current in-home care programs have been roundly criticized for largely ignoring the perspectives of consumers, and caregivers appear to have received even less attention than care recipients when it comes to quality assessment (Applebaum, Straker, & Geron, 2000). As the first phase of a study designed to devise a comprehensive quality management system for family caregiver support services, we sought to learn about quality from those who give and receive caregiver support services.

UNDERSTANDING AND DEFINING QUALITY

Efforts to ensure the quality of services in the aging network have relied heavily on the traditional quality assurance approach. Under this strategy, a series of quality standards are usually developed by state and/or federal funding agencies; these standards are typically based on monitoring and compliance, emphasizing structural and procedural dimensions of a program such as criminal background checks, number of hours of training, and proper record keeping. Providers receive an inspection or monitoring visit and they are informed about their compliance rate. Questions about how their rate of compliance affects consumers, how they compare to other providers, and how they can improve are rarely included in the review process. In most instances the monitoring of standards focuses on a review of agency records. Direct contact with consumers themselves is generally quite limited. Because of the exclusion of consumers and the lack of an overall improvement strategy, critics have suggested that our efforts to ensure and improve quality need to be modified (IOM, 2001; Kane, Kane, & Ladd, 1998). In the case of caregiver support programs, additional complexity occurs with attempts to define the consumer, because both caregivers and care receivers are affected by many of the services such as respite (through adult day services or home care).

The research reported in this chapter was part of a larger Administration on Aging (AoA)–funded project based on the NFCSP in Ohio. Conducted in collaboration with the Ohio Department on Aging and three area agencies on aging, the project focused on the development of NFCSP service quality standards that are caregiver centered and outcomes based. The early stages of the NFCSP implementation provided an ideal situation to design a quality system that avoided some of the problems of the monitoring-focused, regulation-based measures commonly used in long-standing programs.

As the first step in the Ohio NFCSP project, we asked consumers about their definitions of quality. A major challenge at this step was to be sensitive to and clear about who the consumer is. As noted earlier, many caregiver support services directly affect the care receiver. For this reason, we included the voices of multiple stakeholders in the project, but kept the focus on caregivers as the primary consumers.

METHODS

The research question for the first phase was: what are the critical elements of quality as defined by the caregivers and care receivers? Because this question is relatively unexplored and requires depth and intensity of dialogue, a qualitative design was most appropriate. We used focus groups to allow both shared and divergent experiences and perspectives to emerge in the group interview process.

Sample

Eight focus groups of stakeholders (caregivers, care receivers, and caregiver support service providers) were conducted in the state of Ohio, with a total of 52 participants. There was geographic diversity across groups, from rural to urban, covering the four corners and center of the state. Groups were conducted over a 10-week period.

We began with a commitment to conduct focus groups primarily with caregivers but knew it was important to also include care recipients and formal service providers. Sampling for each group was flexible and emergent by design, with the ongoing analysis of the earlier groups informing group composition, questions, and strategies in the later groups. The first four groups were homogeneous by stakeholder type; three of the final four groups were mixed. We began and concluded with all-caregiver groups. Of the 52 participants, 39 were caregivers, 7 were providers, and 6 were care receivers.

Caregiver support services used by participants included information and referral/assistance, transportation, and respite care (in-home and adult day services). For the most part, the groups were heterogeneous by gender, race, age, and care experience; and among caregivers and care receivers, we sought a diversity of caregiver relationships, for example, filial, spousal, and sibling. Caregiver ages ranged from 40 to 94. Care-giving ranged from instrumental, part-time support in separate living ar-rangements, to co-residential, intimate, 24-hour personal care. Duration of care ranged from less than 1 year to more than 17 years. Among caregivers, most were women caring for their husbands, followed by daughters and daughters-in-law, and other relatives. Participants were re-cruited through Area Agencies on Aging and senior centers. Caregiver and care receiver participants received a stipend ($25.00) for their time and contribution.

Data Collection and Analysis

Semistructured interview schedules were constructed to broadly explore four central topics: when support services have made a positive differ-ence in the life of a caregiver, when services (or lack thereof) have had a negative impact on the caregiver, what caregivers hope services will ac-complish for them, and how they know (and we can know) when these goals are accomplished. With the exception of the provider group, each group began by asking participants to briefly describe their care experi-ences and relationships as well as their use of support services. In the rare case when the group dynamic by itself did not cover the four major topics, the interview schedule was used as a default tool. In the provider group, members were asked to identify caregiver needs, service outcomes, and quality indicators.

Each of the focus groups was facilitated by the same researcher. Inter-views were audio recorded and transcribed verbatim. Interview texts were the primary data analyzed; observed nonverbal behaviors and dynamics also informed the analysis. We used an open coding method, refining and revising codes within and across interviews, including a constant compar-ative method. Through this process, we built a conceptual framework for our analysis.

RESULTS

The caregivers, service providers, and care receivers who participated in our focus groups shared with us a range of experiences, emotions, and insights. We asked participants in all groups to tell us about the four cen-tral topics mentioned previously. From these questions, caregivers shared stories covering a wide variety of situations, replete with many issues, concerns, examples, and themes. Overall, the focus groups provided us a picture of the strength, adaptability, courage, struggle, and sacrifice that is part of family caregiving. The need for caregiver support was strongly affirmed by the focus groups. The following quotes from three caregivers help to illustrate the challenge of their roles; these quotes further underscore the importance of developing a system of services that is built on caregiver needs and evaluated based on caregiver outcomes.

> *"It just seems like everything I have is falling away. And she's not financially able to pay out a lot. So, I've kind of sacrificed myself, and . . . you know, to help her."*

> *"My mother's ninety-five. She came to live with us temporarily fourteen years ago."*

> *"We put the monitoring system in her room. Well, she screams so loud that we had to take it out. My husband couldn't get any sleep to go to work. My granddaughter couldn't get any sleep to go to school. I haven't slept in my bed for two and a half years . . . I have to set the alarm every two hours. I have to go and turn her."*

In addition to powerful testimonies that underscore the need for caregiver support services, three major categories of information emerged to help us understand caregivers' conceptions of quality.

1. Quality of life: What do caregivers need to maintain their quality of life?
2. Quality of services: What do services need to do to support caregivers?
3. Quality of the service system: What system organization issues affect the quality of caregiver support?

Quality of Life

Participants helped us understand what was important to them, what they as caregiver needed to have for a good quality of life. These themes can best be summarized as fill-ins for the statement, **To achieve quality of life, I need to:**

Feel OK about myself and my decisions
Participants talked about the need to achieve a sense of peace in their lives and accept the compromises and difficult decisions they have had to make.

Feel OK about the services my care receiver gets
Caregivers discussed the impact of services on their care receiver as a dimension of quality of life. If a worker was coming in to the home, or the care receiver was going to adult day services, it was important

to the caregivers to know that the care receiver was OK with these arrangements.

Keep activities at home as normal as possible
Being able to preserve some sense of a normal or usual everyday life at home was important, including sitting down to dinner, working on homework with kids or grandchildren, and having a conversation.

Continue usual roles as much as possible
Caregivers wanted to maintain their social roles as best they could. They identified the importance of maintaining friendships and other family roles, continuing paid or volunteer work, and continuing activities that they deemed important.

Have true respite (vs. simply time off)
This distinction between time off and a true sense of respite or relief reflects caregivers' need to feel some freedom from the stress and responsibility of caregiving. They made it clear that this sense of relief is not always the same (nor can it be evaluated in the same way) as just getting out of the house or having time away from their care receivers. Further details about true respite are discussed in the section on respite services.

Take care of myself
Caregivers discussed the importance of maintaining their physical and mental health. Having time to be alone was mentioned as important.

Know help is there if and when I need it
Caregivers often were hesitant to use help, but knowing that assistance was available was identified as important.

These revelations about caregivers' definitions of quality of life have explicit implications for specific services and implicit implications for the goals that can underlie the design and delivery of services. For example, knowing that it is important for caregivers to "feel OK about myself and my decisions" can be translated into training tips about communication and interaction for home care workers and information and assistance professionals.

Quality of Services

Caregivers, service providers, and care recipients discussed the ways in which services made life better, or failed to make a positive difference in quality of life. Focus group members were asked specifically about three caregiver support services that are commonly offered under the NFCSP:

Table 9.1 Caregiver Views on Quality of Services

Information and Assistance Support Me When...	Transportation Supports Me When...	"True Respite" Supports Me When...
I have called the one right person (or agency). I feel understood. I am treated with respect and compassion. I get information right away. I get all the information I ask for. I get above and beyond what I ask for. I am not overwhelmed by information. I know what to do next.	I can count on it (it comes and goes on time). It goes where we need to go. It is affordable. It is good for my care receiver. I know my care receiver is safe and comfortable. My care receiver accepts the transportation. The ride is not overlong. The driver demonstrates a caring attitude. The driver goes above and beyond.	Others communicate to me my right to respite, that I deserve a break, that it is normal to need a break. My care receiver accepts or welcomes the respite arrangement. I can count on my break (that it will happen, that it will be uninterrupted). My break is available when I need it most. What I want to happen, happens. My privacy is protected. I know and trust the workers. I believe the workers genuinely care about me and my care receiver. The worker goes above and beyond. The workers know what they are doing. The workers show patience. The workers listen to, respect, and use my input.

information and assistance, transportation, and respite, both in-home and adult day care. Table 9.1 provides a listing of the participants' description of quality for these services. We grouped these responses into the following categories: access to services, timing of assistance, information about the care recipient and his or her services, and worker impact.

Access to Services

Before assessing the quality of a caregiver service, an initial step involves making sure the caregiver and care receiver have access to the assistance needed. This may mean knowing the right person to call for information and assistance, that the transportation service is affordable, or whether there is an adult day care center in the area. Access and affordability are service quality issues. Although most quality assurance efforts don't begin until after someone is enrolled in a particular program, the first step in quality is getting the service to those who need it.

Timing of Assistance

A long-standing criticism of in-home services is that services were delivered when it was convenient for the provider, but not necessarily when it worked for the care recipient and caregiver. A consistent theme discussed by caregivers was the importance of getting the service when they needed it. This was especially true when caregivers discussed the concept of respite. Caregivers who need respite to attend a religious or social function, or for a health care appointment described needing respite on their schedule, not the providers' schedule. Service availability for evenings and weekends has been a longstanding challenge for service providers.

Information About the Care Recipient and His or Her Services

Caregivers discussed the importance of getting the necessary information about service options and also about how the care recipient responded to the services. Being informed was particularly important to caregivers receiving respite services. For example, caregivers described how important it was to them to know about what was happening in the adult day care setting. How was the care recipient doing at the site? Did she seem comfortable and involved? Were there any concerns from the provider perspective? Caregivers indicated that a service was true respite only if it worked for both the caregiver and the care recipient.

Worker Impact

Given the intense relationship shared by the direct care worker, the caregiver, and the care receiver, it is not surprising that many of the quality comments focused on the workers. Whether the service was transportation, information and assistance, personal care, or adult day care, respondents were consistent about their definitions of a quality worker. Trust, respect, caring, listening, and going above and beyond were words commonly used to describe workers and their contributions to the quality of life of caregivers and care recipients. It was clear that the worker is an essential ingredient in the quality formula.

Quality of the Service System

Although we did not explicitly ask focus group participants to share views about the overall system of services (including services for care recipients and those for care receivers), their comments and concerns revealed some complexities in the system that must be considered as we design measures and processes for quality. Following are some of complexities of the system revealed through the focus group discussions.

Caregivers Have a Critical Role in Identifying Success in Program Outcomes

Quality of a caregiver support service begins and ends with the caregiver. The centrality of caregiver voice in defining quality is illustrated in the following statements:

"An outcome is something I am seeking."

"An outcome has been achieved when I say it has."

"Quality is what I say it is."

For a system that has paid limited attention to consumers in general, this focus on caregivers as consumers of services and as experts on the quality of those services represents a significant shift.

Each Caregiver and Family Is Different

Many common themes and issues were discussed across groups and across circumstances, but we also learned about many unique situations. Quality should take into account the variable dynamics, goals, and situations of families and caregivers. Quality can best be understood as the closest fit between what is needed and sought and what is communicated and provided.

The Caregiver Is Part of a Family System

No matter how, why, or to whom we think we are *delivering* services, nearly all services are *received* by families. For example, home-delivered meals are designed, delivered, and assessed as a service to care receivers. However, many caregivers mentioned this service as a source of respite for them. Understanding the impact of any service on the entire family is essential. It is equally important to consider the complementary, competing, or conflicting goals for all family members who are affected by services. Adding to the complexity of services and recipients, it is important to keep in mind that one family may have multiple caregivers and/or multiple care receivers. High-quality services must necessarily be the outcome of well-negotiated family decisions.

Services May Add Stress and Costs

Services induce costs for families, including financial costs, loss of privacy, and loss of control. Services can also introduce or exacerbate stress, especially when the system is confusing, stigmatizing, and intrusive. For services to be regarded as high quality, the value of the service must outweigh its stressors or costs. One focus group member illustrated this point when she said, "Out of the [two-week respite] I may have had three to four days where I could probably put it out of my mind and really try to rest. The rest of the time you're concerned about, you know, what's happening with her."

Services Are Experienced in Stages

Caregivers and families become involved with the service system in stages, including awareness of the service, making an initial contact, initiating service, transitioning into a new kind or new level of service, and terminating the service. Needs and expectations change according to these stages. Each stage has its own quality issues.

Family Circumstances (Functional Health, Resources, Family Composition, and Perspectives) Change

The needs, goals, and expectations of the caregiver and the family change as circumstances change. Because of this dynamic situation, quality systems have to be built to be flexible, so that quality assessment and improvement efforts can accommodate a moving target.

SUMMARY: CAREGIVERS AS CONSUMERS AND AS EXPERTS ON QUALITY

These focus groups provided invaluable insights into understanding quality and its relationship to maintaining care at home. The caregiver stories, their insights, and their challenges helped us to understand the many dimensions and definitions of quality of services and quality of life. Perhaps most importantly, their words helped us to sharpen our focus; they helped us to understand what it really means to focus on caregivers, with all that implies in terms of multiple, mutual, and sometimes conflicting needs and agendas played out in the emotional arena of a family trying to do what is best. Family caregivers have generally been recognized as an important part of the aging network, but they have often been the invisible foundation of the system rather than as active consumers and participants. These focus groups reinforced the fact that caregivers are in the center of the picture, right next to the care recipient.

To integrate this perspective into a quality management model requires answers to very specific questions about the measurement of quality: How is quality defined? What questions are asked to assess quality? Of whom and by whom are these questions asked? How are these data used to improve services? An integrated approach to quality requires a balance among family, individual, and regulatory agendas. An integrated quality model also requires a dialogue among all of the stakeholders in the quality process (families, consumers, providers, and public agency administrators) to identify, formalize, and reinforce new common ground and shared agendas in the definition and measurement of the quality of caregiver support services.

ACKNOWLEDGMENTS

This project was funded by a subcontract from the Ohio Department on Aging as part of Grant 90CG2550 from the Administration on Aging.

REFERENCES

Administration on Aging. (2000). *America's families care: A report on the needs of America's family caregivers.* Washington, DC: U.S. Administration on Aging.

Applebaum, R. A., Straker, J. K., & Geron, S. M. (2000). Assessing satisfaction in health and long-term care: Practical approaches to hearing the voices of consumers. New York: Springer Publishing Company.

General Accounting Office. (1977). *The well-being of older people in Cleveland, Ohio (HRD-77-70).* Washington, DC: U.S. General Accounting Office.

Greene, R., & Feinberg, L. F. (1999). State iniatives for caregivers of people with dementia. *Generations, 23*(3), 75.

Institute of Medicine. (2001). In G. S. Wunderlich & R. O. Kohler (Eds), *Improving the quality of long-term care.* Washington, DC: National Academy Press.

Kane, R. A., & Penrod, J. D. (1995). *Family caregiving in an aging society: Policy perspectives.* Newbury Park, CA: Sage.

Kane, R. A., Kane, R. L., & Ladd, R. (1998). *The heart of long-term care.* New York: Oxford University Press.

Kunkel, S. R., Applebaum, R. A., & Nelson, I. M. (2003–2004). For love and money: Paying family caregivers. *Generations, 27*(4), 74–80.

Levine, C., Reinhard, S. C., Feinberg, L. F., Albert, S., & Hart, A. (2004). Family caregivers on the job: Moving beyond ADLs and IADLs. *Generations, 27*(4), 17.

The Consumer/Provider Relationship as Care Quality Mediator

Barbara Bowers
Sarah L. Esmond
Sally Norton
Elizabeth Holloway

BACKGROUND/SIGNIFICANCE

The Wisconsin Partnership Program (WPP) is a community-based, consumer-centered, comprehensive health and supportive services program for frail elderly and permanently disabled low-income adults. Established with funding from the Robert Wood Johnson Foundation in 1993, the WPP began as a research/demonstration program in Madison, Wisconsin.

This paper describes the findings from formative research conducted during the first 3 years of the program, and focuses on the frail elderly population. Several research initiatives were conducted as the WPP evolved. The specific initiative described here focuses on efforts to define and implement a consumer-centered program.

Although the WPP was committed to a consumer-centered model of care, the absence of an available definition or working model of consumer-centered care made it difficult to proceed with implementing a consumer-centered program. Without such a model, and in the context of considerable disagreement among staff, as well as in the literature, about what consumer-centered care would look like, the program design-ers had little guidance in *how* to design, provide, monitor, or evaluate a consumer-centered program. A review of the literature on consumer-centered care was of limited use. It tended to be highly ideological, con-taining very little practical advice. For example, many of the articles reviewed emphasized the importance of "including" the consumer with-out specifying in practical terms how such inclusion should occur. There was almost nothing in this literature suggesting *how or where* consumers could be effectively included in consumer-centered programs (Lutz & Bowers, 2000). There were also commentaries and studies that identi-fied the nature of choices that consumers in consumer-centered social and support service programs might be offered. But there was almost nothing to guide the Partnership designers in how to provide services or choices in consumer-centered health programs. Defining, implementing, and evalu-ating consumer-centered care became a central goal of the WPP.

To begin the process, prior to program implementation, the research team interviewed a group of frail older adults about their past experiences with health care services and providers. Interviews were also conducted following implementation of the Partnership program and as the program evolved. These interviews provided the research team with important in-sights into how frail elderly consumers thought about their health care, the choices that were important to them, their preferences, and their overall reluctance to express dissatisfaction with services. This paper summarizes what the Partnership research team learned from the interviews with older adults. It raises questions about how to capture the voices of consumers across long-term care settings and identifies barriers to eliciting feedback from frail elders. The insights gained from these interviews were used to design a consumer-centered, highly integrated model of care.

METHODS

A Grounded Dimensional Analysis was selected for the research method (Bowers & Caron, 2000; Schatzman, 1991; Schatzman & Strauss, 1973; Strauss, 1987). This is a variant of the Grounded Theory Method, con-sistent with grounded theory but differing somewhat in the sequenc-ing of analytic procedures. The procedures used in this study follow Schatzman's Dimensional Analysis. The concepts presented in this re-port are derived from the interviews with older adults, rather than im-posed by the researchers. In this sense, the study is grounded in the sub-jects understanding of the phenomenon (in this case how they think about the quality of their care). This report is drawn from a larger study of the Partnership Program implementation and evolution, which also examined provider perspectives, team development, and community integration.

Subjects

Interviews from 75 older adults were used for this report. Subjects were initially drawn from the eligible pool of low income, frail, chronically ill older adults who were enrolled in the PACE program, which preceded the Wisconsin Partnership Program. Later, as the project progressed, more subjects were drawn from Partnership Program enrollees. All older adults who were able to participate in an interview and who consented to an interview were included.

Data Collection

Data collection included formal unstructured interviews with older adults and participant observation in the Partnership Program. Early interviews with consumers were conducted using an open-ended, unstructured interview format. This allowed the subjects to determine the direction of the interviews. Later interviews were more focused, building on analysis completed on previous interview data. Consumers were encouraged to explain and illustrate how they distinguished high-quality care from lesser quality care, to identify the criteria used to make such distinctions, and to illustrate what they looked for and valued in service providers. Interviews were conducted individually with older adults in a place where privacy was assured. Often the researchers met with subjects several times, for very short periods of time because of subject fatigue and illness. The researchers believed it was important to include any subjects willing to participate, despite the challenges of illness and disability. All interviews were audio taped and transcribed for the purpose of analysis. Required human subjects' protocols were filed and approved before any data collection occurred.

Data Analysis

Data were analyzed using Dimensional Analysis (Bowers & Caron, 2000; Schatzman, 1991; Strauss, 1987). The method is consistent with a symbolic interactionist perspective (Shalin, 1986) and was developed by Schatzman. Dimensional analysis involves a line-by-line method of open coding and focuses on how informants/subjects think about the phenomenon (e.g., how they define quality of care). The method also facilitates a comparative analysis of how different groups of subjects (such as consumers vs. providers or across subgroups of consumers) understand care quality and includes differences and similarities in the way each views the topic. Thus, in this study, consistencies and variations in how subjects understood care quality were "discovered" through careful analysis of their accounts of the care they received or watched others receive. Dimensional Analysis is a particularly useful method to explore in areas where there is little known and/or areas in which there are important perspectives missing from our general understanding. Analysis proceeds from a very open to a more focused interview process that allows the researcher to delineate the logic reflected in subjects' descriptions of the phenomenon (care quality). Interviews become more focused as the study evolves.

FINDINGS

Findings from this study suggest that relationships with service providers are extremely important for frail older consumers. Further, the significance of the consumer/provider relationship is both social and highly practical. The implications are that consumers can tell us something about quality that goes well beyond whether the experience was socially pleasant.

It is the practical implications of the consumer/provider relationship that are not generally appreciated and will be the focus of the findings section.

RELATIONSHIP AS MEDIATOR

Integrating the Personal Details With Care and Treatment Decisions

Consumers consistently described how the familiarity resulting from an ongoing relationship with a care provider increased the likelihood of receiving higher quality care and how such familiarity influenced the quality of their care. In particular, they described how a provider's knowledge about a consumer's personal fears and concerns influenced both the provision and the acceptance of care. For example, one older woman described the consequence of her doctor's awareness that she "dreaded" being hospitalized. In discussing the possibility of being admitted to the hospital, she said, "He would never ask me to do that. He knows how nervous it would make me."

She went on to describe that she had three cats at home that she was very attached to and very concerned about. When she was gone for any length of time, she worried incessantly about their well-being. Because her doctor was aware of this concern, he would only hospitalize her, she explained, if there was absolutely no other option. Knowing this, she was willing to go into the hospital only when *he* advised it because she was certain that her doctor had taken her discomfort with the consequences into account. If, however, another doctor suggested that she needed to be admitted to a hospital, she would likely refuse. In this second instance, she explained that her dread of leaving her cats could not have been factored into the decision. This lack of familiarity and understanding left her uncertain about the *real* necessity of hospitalization. Thus, the consumer/provider relationship influenced this subject's willingness to accept her physician's recommendations.

Making the Self Visible

The interviews with older adults also revealed another important consequence of the relationship with their providers. A positive result of a high-quality consumer/provider relationship is an increased likelihood of patient compliance. An important component of the relationship is the ability of a provider to bring the past forward, to see beyond the frailty and decline to the person hidden from view to those who have no shared history or knowledge of the person. One older, retired chemistry professor offered an example of the very high-quality care he had received from a doctor. This doctor always talked with him about the chemistry involved in the drugs that he prescribed for the professor. The professor admitted to feeling better about the care he received from this particular doctor and enjoyed visits to her office. He also suggested that he was much more "compliant" with the prescriptions from that particular physician than he was with others. The chemistry professor talked with pride about this physician who "treats me like an intelligent human being, and not just an old man." Thus, the ability of a provider to bring the self forward, to make the person inside the failing body visible, not only resulted in a higher quality relationship and a more satisfying visit for the patient but also led to a greater likelihood of successful treatment.

Medical/Biographical Expertise

Subjects suggested that when providers had adequate knowledge about their personal *and* medical histories, mistakes were likely to be minimized. Several consumers recounted stories of how this operated in clinical situations. For example, some consumers talked about how frightening it was when a health care provider asked questions about their medical histories. This suggested to consumers that the provider did not have access to important health information. Lacking such access, this meant that the provider was relying on the consumer's memory to make important health decisions. One woman, recounting her visit to a clinic commented, "He didn't have my records with him or hadn't read them. He said, 'Now tell me what drugs you are taking and what you are taking them for?' Well, I knew I was in trouble." Remembering the patient's history or having quick access to the records gave considerable comfort to patients with complicated medical histories. Almost all the older adults interviewed expressed concern over the difficulty they had in remembering important details about their medical histories. The researchers discovered that many providers asked these questions as confirmation, even though they had access to the patients' records and already knew the answers in many cases. These providers were unaware of the unease and burden they generated by asking these questions, or by asking them in a way that suggested the consumer was expected to keep track of the information.

Long-term relationships between consumers and providers also resulted in some providers integrating their knowledge of the consumers' fears and intolerances into a plan of care. For example, one woman revealed that she had a very low intolerance of nausea. She was reluctant to take any medication that left her even slightly nauseated. Her provider was aware of this and, without any intervention or reminders from her, always addressed the possibility of nausea occurring, selecting another medication whenever possible. In some instances, the physician might use "the second best drug" to avoid the possibility of nausea. When he determined that a particular drug was necessary, even though it might cause nausea, he discussed this with the consumer, including what they would do if she began to experience any discomfort. Again, personal knowledge, familiarity, and relationship lead to more technically appropriate, higher quality care and undoubtedly greater compliance with the treatment plan.

What makes this example significant is that many of the older adults interviewed for this study had stopped taking medications that gave them unpleasant side effects. In many of these cases they had not informed their physicians that they had done this. In fact, in several of these situations, the consumers told their physicians that they continued to take the drug. Subjects explained that they were unwilling to inform physicians about untoward drug side effects or that they had decided to stop taking a drug. Some feared that revealing this would make the physician angry. Some feared they would get the physician in trouble. Some believed this was evidence that the physician did not know how the drug worked or what side effects it had. A patient's failure to discuss side effects and reluctance to inform the physician about discontinuing a drug were much more likely to occur if the physician had not informed the patient about the possible side effects.

EVIDENCE FOR CARE QUALITY: THE CONSUMERS' VIEW

Analysis of the consumer interviews also gave insight into the types of evidence consumers use to assess the quality of care they receive. That evidence closely parallels the consumer descriptions of good consumer/provider relationships described previously. For example, consumers identified the importance of evidence that their provider has remembered personal details about them. There was quite a range in both the type of details and the degree to which this type of experience reflected a level of intimacy or familiarity. One older woman, Edith, explained how upsetting it had been when a physician she knew well had referred to her as Ethel. She was suddenly faced with the realization that she did not have the relationship with this provider that she had believed she had. In addition, her concern that "He might be giving me Ethel's medicine" shifted her view of the quality of care that she was currently receiving and would likely receive in the future. In another instance, an older man described how his physician was working with a medical student and had told the student about the man's wife, what his adult children were doing, and how complicated his medical situation was. The details were all recounted accurately. This gave the older man tremendous reassurance that his physician would remember other details that were important to his care.

Some consumers also described how explicitly integrating personal details into care and treatment plans served as evidence of care quality. For example, a woman who was hospitalized explained how her physician made the decision to keep her overnight because of her transportation difficulties *without her reminding him about this*. An older man described how the doctor's actions during clinic visits reflected his understanding of the patient's history: "I know you always get cold, so I'll put a heater in Room Two. You'll have to wait a bit longer, but the room will be warm." This reassured the man that the physician "knew him and his condition." Another informant explained that her physician asked how she would follow her diet while she took care of her young grandchildren, even asking what assistance might be required, revealing intimate knowledge of the patient without the patient reminding her. In each of these cases, consumers described this as evidence of concern *and* competence and how much easier it was to trust the provider, trust the care decisions, and follow the treatment plans.

In contrast to these examples, several consumers talked about how upset and anxious they became when providers forgot important details like those described previously, dismissed them as unimportant, or did not integrate these into a plan of care. Lack of integration of such personal details into treatment plans suggested to consumers that either the provider had forgotten important things about them or simply didn't care. In these situations, consumers were reluctant to remind providers and generally did not report doing so. There was certainly no sense in reminding a provider to consider something that had been dismissed from lack of concern. Many of these latter situations led to consumers simply ignoring the advice and/or treatment plans they had been given, generally without informing the provider that they had done so. The implications for care quality and efficacy are obvious.

Making and/or maintaining eye contact was also widely cited by consumers as evidence of care quality, suggesting that a provider who was more caring was likely to be more attentive, more likely to remember important details, and to integrate important biographical and medical information into the plan of care. In addition to a lack of confidence about the care they would receive, lack of eye contact sometimes resulted in consumers having a decreased willingness to share important information with their providers. Consumers interpreted their providers' absence of eye contact as both a lack of opportunity for disclosing information and an indication that the provider was not listening to them. Thus, the consumer/provider relationship clearly influences the comprehensiveness of information providers have access to and has clear implications for care quality.

Finally, several consumers identified providers' willingness to *clear the way* for them in difficult situations as evidence of *both* a good relationship and a high level of care quality. Several consumers described *clearing the way* as activities physicians (and other providers) engage in that influence the quality and effectiveness of, or the consumer's tolerance for care provided by someone else. For example, a physician might call ahead to make sure another provider is informed about medication intolerances; a physician might call the hospital unit to convey important details about the consumer in order to ensure that knowledge is factored into their care. A physician might also make special requests, such as asking a home health agency to alter their usual routines in order to better accommodate a consumer. Clearing the way increases the likelihood that the care provided by others, in settings other than the doctor's office (hospital staff, specialists, etc.), is of high quality. It is significant that clearing the way can only be done if the provider has both a high level of familiarity with the consumer and is willing to use this knowledge to advocate on behalf of the consumer.

This level of attention to detail was particularly important for consumers who had some sort of unusual circumstance, or whose care deviated in some way from usual practice. Some consumers spoke about ways in which their care requirements were unusual (the rapidity of blood sugar changes, the great significance of a seemingly benign symptom) and the lengths *good* providers would go to convey to others how *this consumer's* care was unique and different.

In many of these instances of *great care*, the providers were engaging in behavior that would legitimize what the consumers would tell others. This increased the likelihood that consumers would be believed. This was particularly important for consumers who had very serious illnesses that could worsen quickly or who had very unusual symptoms.

CONSUMER CHOICES

Consumers were each asked to talk about the things that were most important to them. Many of the responses to this question came from past experiences when consumers had not been allowed to participate in the choices they deemed important. There was considerable consistency among consumers on which choices were most important. Although choice of physician was quite important for almost everyone, choice of personal care worker or home health aide was an even more valued choice for those who had experience with home care or personal care services.

Consumers also identified the timing and scheduling of events as an important area for them to have choices. This desire for choice ranged from when they would see a doctor to what time the personal care worker would arrive. This preference was generally related to very practical issues. For example, one man who was seriously disabled (although younger than most other consumers in the program) described how important it was for his personal care worker to arrive between 7 A.M. and 7:30 A.M. "When he's late, which is quite a lot, I have to decide whether to stay in bed all day or make my wife late for work. You see I'm a two-person transfer." Another subject explained how she had decided not to see her doctor unless it was urgent because the scheduling of transportation was always difficult and generated much anxiety for her.

Consumers also described the importance of the way an organization scheduled workers, how activities/services such as bathing and meals were scheduled, and the difficulty of having the worker determine these activities. Consumers stated that they rarely complained to staff about the lack of choice, despite the significance of these choices for their quality of life. Consumers were quite reluctant to complain for fear of (1) sounding ungrateful, (2) angering the worker or the organization, or (3) becoming frustrated over having unfulfilled expectations. Further, according to consumers, they were unlikely to provide negative or critical feedback even if it were solicited by the worker's agency.

A third important choice identified by consumers concerned the intensity of treatments. This is clearly a choice that relates more to health care than to social services. Consumers consistently expressed distress over their inability to control how aggressively health conditions were treated. In most cases, they described how the treatments had interfered so much with their quality of life that they would stop medications or cut back on dosages without consulting their physician. Among respondents, this altering of treatment plans, on their own, was quite common. In most instances, these consumers felt that they had not been given any choice. In general, they also described considerable pressure to accept treatments without protest and were given little support to alter the treatment when they mentioned the side effects. Instead, in most instances, they described being reminded of how important the treatment was. Some of these consumers suggested that they would have opted out of the treatments altogether. Others said they would have welcomed the option to discuss the treatment and alter it in a way that was less aggressive and had fewer side effects.

Consumers also talked about the importance of being able to choose the side effects they had to live with. Some side effects were simply not tolerated. Others were endured, although they interfered significantly with the consumer's quality of life. It was surprising to the research team how many consumers were no longer taking medications that had been prescribed, even though they had never informed their physicians that they had stopped taking the drug. Having some opportunity to discuss the side effects, and to select the drug that was less likely to cause poorly tolerated side effects, was quite important to consumers. For some, knowing that difficult side effects were a possibility *and* that the drug could be changed if that occurred was sufficient to increase compliance.

The focus of treatment was also considered an important choice and was, again, a choice that consumers felt they rarely had any impact on. This group of consumers tended to have multiple health problems requiring complex treatment plans. In several instances, the providers seemed to be focusing on problems that were less important to the consumers than were other problems that the providers seemed to be ignoring. One woman talked at length about the importance of being able to navigate the five steps into her home while the care provider focused on her heart and kidney problems. The woman was tremendously frustrated as she noted her own slow decline and became very anxious about her ability to stay in her home. The provider expressed little sympathy, suggesting that she should look for a place to live that had no steps. After enrolling in the Partnership Program, the team identified both her kidney problems and her ability to climb the five steps as priorities that required intervention. As a consequence, she became more cooperative with the overall treatment plan and her fear was reduced considerably.

Finally, consumers talked about the importance of deciding where they would live. Whether deciding to stay in their home or selecting a supportive housing environment, consumers unanimously wanted final say in where they went to live, even for a short time. This was reflected in consumer frustration over providers not attending to the health problems that might interfere with living where they wanted to live (such as navigating the five steps).

Evaluating Care Quality: Impact of the Relationship

Consumers were all asked to provide examples of the best and the worst care they had ever received. These descriptions provided interesting insights into how consumers evaluated their care and the dimensions that entered into those evaluations. Some descriptions of *the best* care included instances in which the outcomes were less than the consumer had hoped for or the care was delivered in a way that caused distress or even harm to the consumer. Whether care was assessed as good or bad depended largely on the relationship between the consumer and provider.

Surprisingly, even in those instances where there were serious negative consequences for the consumers, they did not necessarily assess the care as *bad*. Statements such as these were quite common: "It wasn't her fault." "Everyone makes mistakes." "It couldn't be helped." "These things happen sometimes." One woman described undergoing a procedure that should not have been painful, but was.

> The doctor stood by and the nurse was very, very helpful through the whole thing. She kinda talked me through it 'cause it hurt so bad and was really, really good to me. And they were there too when I had to have my leg up with that sandbag on for eight hours at a time and it wasn't their fault that the thing started bleeding again . . . but they were very, very kind to me, both the nurses and the doctors. So I'd say that was one time that I had really good care.

When asked about such instances, the explanations consumers gave were often focused on the *intent of the provider than on the provider's competence or the outcome*. For example, in one situation where a consumer experienced a serious negative, preventable outcome, she prefaced the description with "Maybe that wasn't supposed to happen, but I know she means well. She really tried." In fact, in many instances, providers were forgiven and care was assessed as high quality based on the consumers' perceptions of the providers' intent:

> "And I told that to the doctor, and she was so sympathetic about it, that I couldn't believe my ears, that she was telling me such kind things and she was so sympathetic that it was just unreal ... And then when she left she had me come into her office to talk to her, and the tears came to my eyes and I just cried and I told her she's the best doctor in the world."

> "I mean, they did the best they could. And they were concerned. They had that ... an attitude that was concerned, you know, that made me feel better to know that they were taking good care of me."

> "I can't remember what he said but what he said made you think he was concerned about how I felt. It was the touch and the attitude that he was doing the best he could."

Conversely, in situations where a consumer did not have a previous positive relationship with a provider in question, assessments were more likely to express negative judgments about the competence of the provider. In those instances where consumers were upset about negative outcomes, they often attributed those outcomes to a lack of concern or attention from the provider rather than to technical inability. This belief seemed to be based on an assumption that differences in provider performance were generated from differences in provider caring. That is, providers who *cared enough* to make sure care was provided in an effective manner would thus provide higher quality care. Consumers gave many examples of how a caring attitude led to care processes (and higher quality) that substantially differed from care given by an unfamiliar or uncaring provider.

In addition to focusing on intent, consumers were seen to minimize the negative consequences, resulting in a more positive overall evaluation of the experience than would be expected. For example, a consumer who had been interviewed in the clinic and was later interviewed in a nursing home described her experience. She had just spoken at length about the importance to her of being walked each day so that she would be able to recover and go home. She then went on to say that she had not been walked for several days in a row. She summed up her experience by saying, "Well, I don't always get my walk, but it's OK. I guess I don't really need it. Maybe other people need it more than I do. I guess it doesn't really matter so much if I get it. There are other things that are more important." She was minimizing the significance of her walks in relation to her overall care as well as minimizing the significance of her care in relation to other residents' care.

DISCUSSION

The relationship between health care provider and consumer has often been talked about as if it were largely irrelevant to the technical quality of the care provided, as *just* part of the amenities. Findings from this study reveal that relationship is much more relevant to care quality than is suggested by these discussions. Consumer assessments of care quality were often embedded in consumers' beliefs about the nature of the relationship they had with the provider. Most importantly, however, this study suggests that the quality and continuity of these relationships affects the technical quality of care patients receive and the willingness of consumers to share pertinent information and follow a recommended treatment plan.

ACKNOWLEDGMENTS

Support for this research provided by the Robert Wood Johnson Foundation, Building Health Systems Initiative Grant 23246.

REFERENCES

Bowers, B. J., & Caron, C. (2000). Methods and application of dimensional analysis: A contribution to concepts and knowledge development in nursing. In L. Rodgers & K.A. Knafl (Eds.), *Concept development in nursing: Foundations, techniques, and applications* (2nd ed., pp. 285–319). Philadelphia: Saunders.

Lutz, B. J., & Bowers, B. J. (2000). Patient-centered care: Understanding its interpretation and implementation in health care. *Scholarly Inquiry for Nursing Practice, 14*(2), 165–183; discussion 183–167.

Schatzman, L. (1991). Dimensional analysis: Notes on an alternative approach to the grounding of theory in qualitative research. In D. R. Maines (Ed.), *Social organizations and social process: Essays in honor of Anselm Strauss* (pp. 303–314). New York: Aldine De Gruyter.

Schatzman, L., & Strauss, A. (1973). *Field research strategies for a natural society.* Englewood Cliffs, NJ: Prentice Hall.

Shalin, D.N. (1986). Pragmatism and social interactionism. *American Sociological Review, 51*(February), 9–29.

Strauss, A. (1987). *Qualitative analysis for social scientists.* New York: Cambridge University Press.

CHAPTER ELEVEN

Resident Satisfaction with Independent Living Facilities in Continuing Care Retirement Communities

Farida K. Ejaz
Dorothy Schur
Kathleen Fox

INTRODUCTION AND BACKGROUND

The issue of consumer satisfaction with care and services becomes critical, given the burgeoning of various types of housing options for the elderly. Many of these housing options, especially continuing care retirement communities (CCRCs) offer a model of long-term care that encompasses a philosophy of providing services and amenities to older residents that adapt to their changing needs across their life span. The central feature of a CCRC is that it guarantees lifetime access to housing and health care in return for an upfront "buy-in" cost and a fixed monthly fee (Krout, Moen, Holmes, Oggins, & Bowen, 2002). Residents may thus age in place without fear of being unable to obtain or afford care and without having to move or be dependent on their family (Krout et al.). Geared toward more affluent elderly people in general, such CCRCs are designed to provide independence and control over one's own destiny (Wylde, 2001).

Because there is wide variation in what elderly consumers desire, understanding and measuring consumer opinions has become a powerful tool that leads to the development of services that are geared to address consumer needs. Such an approach focuses on the creation of client-centered service delivery (Moran, White, Eales, Fast, & Keating, 2002). Recognition of the advantages to consumer-directed care has led many long-term care providers to use consumer satisfaction surveys. However, a major criticism of such surveys is that these instruments have not been tested for their reliability and validity (Cohen-Mansfield, Ejaz, & Werner, 2000). Another criticism is that satisfaction is examined in isolation and lacks conceptual and empirical clarity (Moran et al.).

This chapter draws on data from a larger study on satisfaction of family members and residents who resided in assisted living and independent living units located in eight Ohio CCRCs (Ejaz, Schur, & Fox, 2003). This chapter focuses exclusively on the satisfaction of residents residing in independent living facilities located within CCRCs because in the long-term care satisfaction literature little attention has been paid to the perspectives of residents who are fairly active and independent. On the other hand, there is an emerging body of literature on satisfaction of nursing home residents (Sangl, 2005; Straker, Ejaz, McCarthy, & Jones, 2005; Wheatley et al., 2005) and assisted living residents (Hawes, Phillips, & Rose, 2000; Rose & Pruchno, 1998). Further, this chapter addresses the two major criticisms of the types resident satisfaction surveys listed previously by (1) testing the psychometric properties of a measure on resident satisfaction in independent living (IL) developed and used by the HealthRays Alliance (HRA), a consortium of 15 non-profit long-term care providers in northeast Ohio; and (2) developing and testing a conceptual model of key issues that are likely to be related to resident satisfaction.

Because a significant piece of the study was to explore the utility of a conceptual model, investigators examined the long-term care literature to identify resident and facility characteristics that were likely to predict overall satisfaction with services and amenities. With respect to resident characteristics, investigators found that *sociodemographic characteristics* such as age, educational levels, and length of stay were likely to influence consumer satisfaction in long-term care settings (Aharony & Strasser, 1993; Cleary et al., 1991; Kruzich, Clinton, & Kelber, 1992). Other resident characteristics that were likely to affect satisfaction included *health and function* variables such as physical and mental health (depression; Mitchell & Kemp, 2000; Namazi, Eckert, Kahana, & Lyon,

1989; Pearlman & Uhlmann, 1988); activities of daily living scores or ADLs (Gould, 1992); *special resources* including social support (Kahn, 1994) and interactions with others including staff (Bitzan & Kruzich, 1990; Faulk, 1988; Kruzich et al., 1992); and *expectations of services*, which includes the perceived importance of services offered and expectations of service quality (Parasuraman, Zeithaml, & Berry, 1986). With respect to *facility characteristics*, the correlates were more difficult to assess because the literature in the area was scant and varied. However, there was literature to suggest that whether a facility was proprietary or nonprofit was likely to influence quality and levels of staffing (Brannon, Zinn, Mor, & Davis, 2002; CDC/NCHS, 1999).

Drawing from this literature, investigators then developed a conceptual model (see Figure 11.1) by extracting key elements from the literature that are likely predictors of resident satisfaction. The model included variables associated with measuring how resident characteristics, health and function, social resources, and expectations of services were likely to predict consumer satisfaction, taking into account whether the IL unit was associated with a for profit or nonprofit CCRC. Prior to testing the conceptual model to examine the predictors of resident satisfaction, investigators examined the psychometric properties of the HRA IL Resident Satisfaction Instrument to ensure that they had a reliable and valid outcome measure of resident satisfaction.

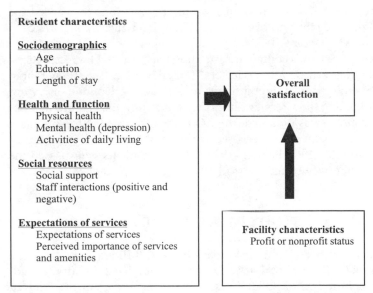

Figure 11.1   Conceptual Model of Consumer Satisfaction in Independent Living.

METHODOLOGY

Selection of Sites

The study's original sample was comprised of CCRCs belonging to HRA. Eight of the 12 CCRCs that were part of HRA agreed to participate. A decision was made to use 2 of these as pilot sites, leaving 6 HRA sites in the study. Investigators recruited 2 non-HRA sites that were for profit CCRCs to add some proprietary facilities to their sample. This article focuses on the findings from the 8 sites (excluding the 2 pilot sites) that participated in the study. Of these 8 sites, 4 CCRCs were located in the suburbs, 3 were urban facilities, and 1 was in a rural area, adding a geographic mix to the participating sites. Six of the 8 facilities were religiously affiliated. All but 2 of the CCRCs were non-profit, and 3 of the 8 were part of a chain.

Study Procedures and Selection of Sample/Respondents

The Institutional Review Board (IRB) mandated that sites receive prior consent from residents to have their names released to the research institute. Based on this approach, sites mailed an introductory letter (drafted by the research institute and IRB approved) explaining the purpose of the study to their residents. This letter stated that residents should notify their CCRC within a 2-week time frame if they did not want their name released to research staff. After the waiting period, sites forwarded the names of all residents who had not refused to have their names released to researchers.

Once the resident's contact information was received by researchers, it was then forwarded to interviewers. Interviewers called the potential respondents to set up an appointment to conduct a telephone interview. Prior to beginning the interview, informed consent to participate was obtained. If consent was obtained, the interviewer proceeded to conduct a cognitive screen using the criteria set by the Short Portable Mental Status Questionnaire (SPMSQ; Pfeiffer, 1975). Those residents who passed the screen were interviewed for the study.

STUDY PARTICIPANTS

Researchers obtained contact information for 158 IL residents from the participating CCRCs. A total of 116 residents completed the survey, leading to a response rate of 73%. Thus, 42 residents were not interviewed from the original list of 158 residents because they refused to participate

(39), could not be contacted on the phone (1), were hard of hearing (1), or could not complete the interview despite passing the cognitive screen (1). The interviews took between 30 and 45 minutes.

Background Characteristics of the Residents

The residents in the study were primarily Caucasian (99%) and female (73%) with a mean age of 82. The majority of them were widowed (59%), whereas 29% of the respondents were married, 10% were single, and 3% were divorced or separated. Forty-one percent had completed college or graduate school, whereas another 26% had attended some college courses. These older adults had resided in their respective units for an average of 3.9 years. They viewed themselves as being physically healthy, rating their health as either very good (38%) or good (45%).

Residents were highly functional with respect to their ADLs. The majority of elders were capable of performing ADLs such as walking (81%), going shopping (78%), preparing meals (89%), taking a bath or shower (96%), getting in and out of bed (100%), and taking care of their appearance (100%) without any help. With respect to how much their physical health interfered with their ability to do things for themselves, 47% believed that their physical health did not interfere at all, whereas another 48% believed it interfered somewhat with their ability to do things for themselves.

Testing a Measure of Consumer Satisfaction in IL Facilities for Reliability and Validity

Prior to testing the conceptual model, investigators examined the psychometric properties of the HRA IL Resident Satisfaction Instrument. The measure had been developed by the administrative staff of HRA with the help of the investigators. The instrument was used to collect consumer satisfaction data and was implemented annually by an external research/consulting firm. The data were then used for quality improvement and for benchmarking purposes. However, the psychometric properties of the instrument had never been systematically tested.

A total of 58 items pertaining to satisfaction with services and amenities comprised the HRA IL Resident Satisfaction measure. In the first step, investigators deleted items with high missing data (15% or more) and the remaining variables (48) were entered into a hierarchical factor analysis (Schmid & Leiman, 1957; Thompson, 1990). This type of hierarchical factor structure analysis is considered appropriate when investigators believe that the implicit design includes a second-order underlying overall measure of a construct as well as first-order solution comprised of specific areas/domains.

The analysis resulted in a first-order 7-factor solution of various domains of satisfaction along with a second-order general factor, or an Overall Satisfaction domain consisting of 48 items. An inclusion and exclusion criteria of .35 was used for the factor loadings in a particular domain/factor. The 6 factors/domains were (1) Admissions, (2) Physical Environment, (3) Dining and Food, (4) Safety and Security, (5) Maintenance of Facility, and (6) Management of Facility. A seventh factor, Helpfulness and Friendliness of Staff and Residents, was dropped because it contained 2 items that investigators believed were not conceptually related; 1 item pertained to helpfulness of food service staff, and the other item referred to the friendliness of residents.

The second-order or Overall Satisfaction domain included all the items identified in the various domains plus 15 additional items for a total of 48 items. In the next step, the aforementioned 6 factors along with the overall satisfaction factor were developed into scales. Reliability of the scales was assessed using Cronbach's alpha and ranged from .76 to .90 (see Table 11.1).

Next, two other questions were treated as outcome variables. One was a single-item measure referring to overall quality of services and amenities (with five response categories ranging from "very good" to "very poor"), whereas the other item focused on the resident's willingness to recommend the facility to other family members and friends (with four response categories ranging from "definitely yes" to "definitely no").

Validity of the six scales as well as the Overall Satisfaction measure was established by running a Pearson Product Correlation between the scales and the two outcome variables. Correlation of the scales with the two outcome variables was all statistically significant. The correlation of the scales with the two outcome variables are listed in Table 11.2.

Testing the Conceptual Model on Resident Satisfaction With IL

Measures Used in the Conceptual Model

Age was measured in years (rounded to the nearest age). Education was measured by five response categories ranging from whether the respondent had completed 0 to 8 years of school to having a master's degree or higher. Length of stay was measured by 10 response categories ranging from less than 1 year to 11 or more years in the facility. Physical health was measured by asking a respondent to rate his or her physical health in comparison to others their age. Depression was measured by the 11-item Center

Table 11.1 Results From the Hierarchical Factor Analysis Using the HRA IL Resident Satisfaction Instrument

Variables	Factor Weights	Alphas
Domain: Admissions		.90
Information you received concerning the services and amenities when you moved in?	.46	
Information on where everything was located?	.52	
Information on who different staff members were?	.51	
Information on how to get services?	.39	
Information about the monthly charges?	.37	
Courtesy and helpfulness of the marketing staff?	.36	
Overall move-in process?	.53	
Domain: Physical environment		.81
Appearance of the grounds?	.67	
Appearance of the buildings?	.73	
Maintenance of sidewalks?	.37	
Overall appearance of the facility and grounds?	.61	
Cleanliness of the facility?	.37	
Domain: Dining and food		.89
Taste of the food?	.55	
Appearance of the food?	.57	
Variety of menu items?	.52	
Food choices as being healthy?	.37	
Temperature of the food?	.51	
Overall quality of the dining services?	.48	
Domain: Safety and security		.76
Safety and security of the living area?	.56	
Safety and security of the facility and grounds?	.53	
Confidence in the facility's response to a medical emergency?	.55	
Domain: Maintenance of facility		.90
Maintenance of the building?	.35	
Process for handling work requests?	.55	
Timeliness of maintenance services?	.61	
Courtesy and helpfulness of the maintenance staff?	.44	
Overall quality of maintenance services?	.46	
Satisfaction regarding decision to move to facility?	.35	
Domain: Management of facility		.90
Concern of the management staff toward resident well-being?	.55	
How well the management staff listens to residents?	.60	
Process for handling resident concerns and requests?	.49	
Reputation of the facility?	.39	
Communication about facility issues?	.54	
Overall management of the facility?	.48	

(continued)

Table 11.1 (Continued)

Variables	Factor Weights	Alphas
Domain: Overall satisfaction (G factor)		.87
Includes all of the above listed variables in addition to the variables listed below.		
Lighting in the grounds?	.58	
Maintenance of streets within the complex?	.60	
Availability of parking?	.53	
Availability of information about emergency procedures (for fire, tornado and other emergencies)?	.57	
Courtesy and helpfulness of the housekeeping staff, in general?	.63	
Overall quality of the housekeeping services?	.67	
Dining room environment?	.67	
Courtesy and helpfulness of food service's staff?	.59	
Variety of activities to reflect your interests?	.57	
Quality of information in the resident handbook?	.77	
Friendliness of the staff?	.60	
Friendliness of the other residents?	.39	
Freedom to live your own lifestyle?	.56	
Feeling of being welcomed when you move into this facility?	.67	
Overall quality of life?	.69	

for Epidemiological Studies Depression Scale (Kohout, Berkman, Evans, & Coroni-Huntley, 1993). ADLs were measured by a 7-item scale that included the extent to which a respondent could perform both physical activities like dressing and bathing, and instrumental activities like grocery shopping or preparing meals (Older American Resources and Services,

Table 11.2 Correlations of Scales With Two Outcome Variables

	Outcome Variables	
Scale	Overall Quality of Services and Amenities	Recommend CCRC to Family and Friends
Admissions	.54***	.49***
Physical environment	.41***	.18*
Dining and food	.49***	.44***
Safety and security	.37***	.23**
Maintenance of facility	.53***	.38***
Management of facility	.56***	.42***
Overall satisfaction	.66***	.50***

*p < .05
**p < .01
***p < .001.

1987). Social support was measured by 7 items and included items such as whether the resident had someone to help if he or she was confined to bed, and someone to share their worries and fears with (adapted from Sherbourne & Stewart, 1991). Staff Interactions was a 7-item measure that captured both positive and negative interactions (Noelker & Poulshock, 1984). Expectations of Services was a 12-item measure and asked residents the extent to which services such as maintenance, dining, programs, and activities had met their expectations after moving to the CCRC. Perceived Importance of Services and Amenities was an 11-item measure that asked respondents to rate the importance of a variety of services offered by a typical CCRC (see Table 11.3 for further details on the measures).

The variables in the model were treated as independent variables, with the outcome variable being the 48-item measure of Overall Satisfaction (G factor). However, prior to running the analyses, a correlation matrix was used to examine all the variables in the model. Using an exclusionary criterion of a correlation of .40 and above between independent variables, investigators dropped 3 items from the conceptual model. These were physical health (this was significantly correlated at .45 with depression), depression (this was significantly correlated at −.45 with activities of daily living), and social support (this was significantly correlated at .50 with perceived importance of services and amenities).

The remaining seven independent variables were entered simultaneously in a multiple regression and included resident demographics, Activities of Daily Living, and Perceived Importance of Services and Amenities. One facility characteristic, whether the CCRC was forprofit or non-profit, was also entered. The final model was significant and had an adjusted R^2 of .27($F = 6.76$; $p < .001$). Only two variables were significant predictors of Overall Satisfaction: (1) Staff Interactions with Residents and (2) Perceived Importance of Services and Amenities (see Table 11.4).

SUMMARY, DISCUSSION, AND IMPLICATIONS FOR PRACTICE

The residents in our study were fairly active and healthy individuals who rated their physical health as being very good or good compared to other people their age. They also did not appear to have problems with depression.

Investigators of this study were able to establish the reliability and validity of the HRA Independent Living Resident Satisfaction instrument. This instrument demonstrated good reliability and validity and had six major domains as well as an Overall Satisfaction measure comprising 48 items.

Table 11.3 Measures in Conceptual Model

Variables	Mean or Percentage	SD	Response Categories	Range	Alpha**
Age	82.32	6.39		57–98	
Education	2.26	1.11	• Grade school or less • Some high school or high school graduate • Some college • Completed college • Master's degree or higher	0–4	
Length of stay in facility	3.91	3.20	• Less than 1 year • 1 to 2 years • 2 to 3 years • 3 to 4 years • 4 to 5 years • 5 to 6 years • 6 to 7 years • 7 to 8 years • 8 to 11 years • 11 or more years	0–9	
Physical health compared to others of the same age	2.21	.73	• Poor • Fair • Good • Very good	0–3	
Mental health	2.48	2.77	• Hardly ever or never • Sometimes • Most of the time	0–2	.78
Activities of daily living*	1.80	.31	• Completely unable • With some help • Without any help	0–2	.78
Social support*	1.72	.41	• Hardly ever or never • Sometimes • Most of the time	0–2	.84
Staff interactions	13.20	1.83	• Hardly ever or never • Sometimes • Most of the time	0–2	.83
Expectations of care	29.52	8.77	• Did not have any expectations • Definitely did not meet expectations • Somewhat met expectations • Definitely met expectations	0–3	.97
Perceived importance of services and amenities*	1.78	.26	• Not at all important • Somewhat important • Very important	0–2	.82

*Mean substitution used in calculating score.
**Alphas based on scores.

Table 11.4   Predictors of Overall Satisfaction

Variables in the Regression	Unstandardized Coefficient (b)	Standardized Coefficient (β)
Staff interaction with resident	.007	.357**
Perceived importance of services and amenities	.360	.232*
Activities of daily living score	.130	.101
Resident expectations of care	.003	.059
Educational level of the resident	.009	.026
Length of time resident has lived in the facility	.003	.023
Age of the resident	−.007	−.102

Note: Final model: adjusted $R^2 = .27$ ($F = 6.76$; $p < .001$).
*$p < .01$.
**$p < .001$.

With respect to testing the conceptual model of consumer satisfaction and identifying the predictors of Overall Satisfaction in CCRCs, this study found that residents placed a high value on their interactions with staff. Our findings revealed that the more positive the interaction between staff and residents, the more satisfied the residents are likely to be. Residents used descriptive phrases such as "friendliness of staff," "their helpfulness," and "employees are very, very kind" to describe their encounters with staff members. It was interesting that such high-functioning and independent residents also place importance on staff–resident interactions. These findings are similar to satisfaction studies conducted with various types of consumers in different long-term care settings. For example, in the historical study that formed the basis of the Omnibus Reconciliation Act of 1987, nursing home residents placed a high value on warm and caring staff (National Citizens' Coalition for Nursing Home Reform, 1985). Similarly, studies of family satisfaction have also found that a negative interaction with staff was the strongest predictor of family satisfaction with care in nursing homes (Ejaz, Noelker, Schur, Whitlatch, & Looman, 2002). In another study, the amount of time that families spent in communicating with staff was a strong predictor of family dissatisfaction (Straker & Ejaz, 2003). In focus groups conducted with residents and family members of assisted living facilities, staffing issues were identified as a major component of quality (Greene, Hawes, Wood, & Woodsong, 1998).

The findings from our study also revealed that understanding what is important to residents is critical to providing services that are responsive to their needs. It suggests that administration and staff need to understand which services are important to residents and make the distinction between what residents desire and what others believe residents *should* be provided with. One resident said, "[Management needs to] talk to residents more," whereas another emphasized the importance of "Better communications between residents and management." Therefore, to provide services that are appropriate and enhance consumer satisfaction, administrators need to encourage positive interaction and communication between residents and staff and continuously seek to discover what residents desire.

Limitations of the Study

The study limitations include the fact that it was conducted in only one state with a small sample of IL residents drawn from eight CCRCs that were predominantly non-profit and were not randomly chosen. The conceptual model was developed from the empirical literature and needs to be further tested and refined. Therefore, to enhance the generalizability of the findings, we recommend the study be replicated with a larger, more representative sample of sites and residents drawn from multiple states. The data from this study can be viewed as initial research findings that provide valuable insights to examine predictors of resident satisfaction in independent living facilities. Future studies need to be conducted with larger, more generalizable samples to verify the information from this project and to examine similarities and differences in consumer satisfaction across the continuum of long-term care settings.

ACKNOWLEDGMENTS

This project was funded by the AARP Andrus Foundation: January 1, 2001, to June 30, 2003. Our thanks to the Continuing Care Retirement Communities that participated in the project: Breckenridge Village, Park Vista Retirement Community, Westminster-Thurber, Brookwood Community, Westview Manor, New Dawn Health Care and Retirement Center, the Renaissance, Rockynol Retirement Community, Laurel Lake Retirement Community, and Mount Pleasant Retirement Village. Our thanks also to James Jones, Director, University Computing Services at Ball State University in Muncie, Indiana; and Shobhana Swami, graduate assistant.

REFERENCES

Aharony, L., & Strasser, S. (1993). Patient satisfaction: What we know about and what we still need to explore. *Medicare Care Review, 50*(1), 352–382.

Bitzan, J. E., & Kruzich, J. M. (1990). Interpersonal relationships of nursing home residents. *The Gerontologist, 30*(3), 385–390.

Brannon, D., Zinn, J. S., Mor, V., & Davis, J. (2002). An exploration of job, organizational, and environmental factors associated with high and low nursing assistant turnover. *The Gerontologist, 42*(2), 159–168.

CDC/NCHS (1999). National Nursing Home Survey. Retrieved April 18, 2005, from www.cdc.gov/nchs/data/nnhsd/NNHS99Employees_selectedchar.pdf.

Cleary, P. D., Edgman-Levitan, S., Roberts, M., Moloney, T., McMullen, W., Walker, J., & Delbanco, T. (1991). Patients evaluate their hospital care: A national survey. *Health Affairs, 278*(19), 254–267.

Cohen-Mansfield, J., Ejaz, F. K., & Werner, P. (Eds.). (2000). *Satisfaction surveys in long-term care.* New York: Springer.

Ejaz, F. K., Noelker, L. S., Schur, D., Whitlatch, C. J., & Looman, W. J. (2002). *Family* satisfaction with nursing home care for relatives with dementia. *Journal of Applied Gerontology, 2*(3), 368–384.

Ejaz, F. K., Schur, D., & Fox, K. (2003). *Consumer satisfaction in continuing care retirement communities.* Final Report to the AARP Andrus Foundation.

Faulk, L. (1988). Quality of life factors in board and care homes for the elderly: A hierarchical model. *Adult Foster Care Journal, 2*(2), 100–117.

Gould, M. (1992). Nursing home elderly: Social environmental factors. *Journal of Gerontological Nursing, 18*(8), 13–20.

Greene, A., Hawes, C., Wood, M., & Woodsong, C. (1998). How do families define quality in assisted living facilities? *Generations, 21*(4), 34–36.

Hawes, C., Phillips, C. D., & Rose, M. (2000). *High service or high privacy assisted living facilities, their residents and staff: Results from a national survey.* Report on A National Study of Assisted Living for the Frail Elderly. Washington, DC: U.S. Department of Health and Human Services.

Kahn, R. (1994). Social support: Content, causes and consequences. In R. Abeles, H. Gift, & M. Ory (Eds.), *Aging and quality of life* (pp. 163–184). New York: Springer.

Kohout, F. J., Berkman, L. F., Evans, D. A., & Coroni-Huntley, J. (1993). Two shorter forms of the CES-D depression symptoms index. *Journal of Aging and Health, 5*(2), 179–193.

Krout, J. A., Moen, P., Holmes, H. H., Oggins, J., & Bowen, N. (2002). Reasons for relocation to a continuing care retirement community. *The Journal of Applied Gerontology, 21*(2), 236–256.

Kruzich, J. M., Clinton, J. F., & Kelber, S. T. (1992). Personal and environmental influences on nursing home satisfaction. *The Gerontologist, 32,* 342–350.

Mitchell, J. M., & Kemp, B. J. (2000). Quality of life in assisted living homes: A multidimensional analysis. *Journal of Gerontology, Psychological Sciences, 55B*(2), 117–127.

Moran, L., White, E., Eales, J., Fast, J., & Keating, N. (2002). Evaluating consumer satisfaction in residential continuing care settings. *Journal of Aging & Social Policy, 14*(2), 85–109.

Namazi, K., Eckert, J., Kahana, E., & Lyon, S. (1989). Psychological well-being of elderly board and care home residents. *The Gerontologist, 29*(4), 511–516.

National Citizens' Coalition for Nursing Home Reform. (1985). *A consumer perspective: The residents' point of view.* Washington, DC: Author.

Noelker, L. S., & Poulshock, S. W. (1984). Intimacy: Factors affecting its development among members of a home for the aged. *International Journal of Aging and Human Development, 19*, 177–190.

Older American Resources and Services. (1987). The OARS multidimensional functional assessment questionnaire: ADL and IADL Sections. In I. McDowell & C. Newell (Eds.), *Measuring health: A guide to rating scales and questionnaires* (pp. 299–306). New York: Oxford University Press.

Parasuraman, A., Zeithaml, V., & Berry, L. L. (1986). *Servqual: A multiple-item scale for measuring customer perceptions of service quality.* Cambridge, MA: Marketing Science Institute.

Pearlman, R., & Uhlmann, R. (1988). Quality of life in chronic diseases: Perceptions of elderly patients. *Journal of Gerontology: Medical Sciences, 43*, M25–M30.

Pfeiffer, E. (1975). A short portable mental status questionnaire for the assessment of organic brain deficit in elderly patients. *Journal of the American Geriatrics Society, 23*(10), 433–441.

Rose, M. S., & Pruchno, R. A. (1998, November). *Residents' and family members' expectations and satisfaction in assisted living.* Poster presentation at the annual meeting of the Gerontological Society of America, Philadelphia, PA.

Sangl, J. (2005). *The development of a CAHPS instrument for nursing home residents (NHCAHPS).* Manuscript submitted for publication.

Schmid, J., & Leiman, J. (1957). The development of hierarchical factor solutions. *Psychometrika, 22*, 53–61.

Sherbourne, C. D., & Stewart, A. L. (1991). The MOS social support survey. *Social Science Medicine (Great Britain), 32*(6), 713–714.

Straker, J., Ejaz, F. K., McCarthy, K., & Jones, J. (2005). *Developing and testing a satisfaction survey for nursing home residents: The Ohio experience.* Manuscript submitted for publication.

Straker, J., & Ejaz, F. K. (2003, November). *Keeping the customer satisfied: Correlates of family satisfaction with Ohio nursing homes.* Symposium presented at the 56th annual conference of the Gerontological Society of America, San Diego, CA.

Thompson, B. (1990). SECONDOR: A program that computes a second-order principal components analysis and various interpretation aids. *Educational and Psychological Measurement, 50*, 575–580.

Wheatley, M. V., Hirsch, M., Walley, J., Lee, C., Urman, H., & Uman, G. (2005). *Implementation and results of the statewide Ohio nursing home resident satisfaction survey.* Manuscript submitted for publication.

Wylde, M. (2001). Independence and satisfaction: What's the connection for independent living and assisted living residents? *Assisted Living Today, November/December,* 43–45.

PART III

Policy Issues and Moral and Legal Challenges

CHAPTER TWELVE

Common or Uncommon Agendas:

Consumer Direction in the Aging and Disability Movements

Robyn I. Stone

INTRODUCTION

Over the past decade, consumer direction in long-term care has received increasing attention by the consumer, practice, and policy communities. A number of factors, including aggressive advocacy by younger people with disabilities, a growing consumer movement in health and long-term care, concerns about the costs of services, and a severe worker shortage, have all contributed to this heightened interest in consumer direction (Stone, 2000).

This chapter addresses the issues related to consumer direction in the aging and disability movements. It begins by defining this concept, highlighting the pivotal role of choice and empowerment, and describing the range of options under the rubric of consumer direction. This is followed by a brief history of the evolution of consumer direction, underscoring the key role of several disability movements and the transfer of this philosophy to the aging services community. The next section identifies the merits and challenges of consumer direction and how these differentially affect various subgroups of people with disabilities. The chapter concludes with some thoughts on the future of consumer direction.

DEFINING CONSUMER DIRECTION

As policymakers, providers, and researchers begin to explore the potential and pitfalls of consumer direction in long-term care, it is critical to provide a clear definition of the concept and to identify the parameters of this approach. Consumer direction is based on the philosophy that individuals with long-term care needs should be empowered to make decisions about the services and supports they receive, including having primary control over the nature of the services and who, when, and how services are delivered.

Consumer direction also assumes that long-term care is predominantly nonmedical, low-tech services and supports that allow individuals with disabilities to function as independently as possible. Thus, the consumer should not be forced to rely on professionals to make key decisions about care and to be "managed" by a formal system.

Consumer direction reflects a continuum of approaches based on the level of decision making, control, and autonomy allowed in a particular situation. At one end of the spectrum, the cash model offers the consumer the most flexibility and potential for empowerment. The consumer decides how to best use the dollars (e.g., purchasing services from a formal vendor, hiring a relative or friend to provide personal care, purchasing some type of assistive device to enhance independence, or modifying one's home to make it possible to remain in the community). Professionally managed service packages, the typical approach used by publicly funded home and community-based care programs, are at the other end (at the less flexible, less empowering end) of the consumer-direction continuum. Even within this approach, however, there is potential for consumer involvement in the development of the care plan and how services are delivered.

Many approaches lie between these two extremes. These range from programs that allow individuals to hire and fire their own workers, to others that allow consumers to hire family members, to voucher programs that, with certain constraints, afford consumers great flexibility in how and where benefits can be used. Other options such as caregiver or disability tax credits also represent a form of consumer direction because they compensate consumers for resources spent (formally or informally) on services and supports. These latter options support the philosophy of consumer direction by providing tax relief when consumers are receiving assistance from, and directly paying, a worker of their choosing

Although consumer direction is considered primarily in the context of home care and personal assistance services, it would be a mistake to dismiss its potential in congregate settings. Small group homes for people with mental retardation and developmental disabilities, for example, provide opportunities for consumer direction for individuals and their families. The underlying philosophy of assisted living is based on the premise that the resident is empowered with significant decision-making authority. Even in the nursing home, it is possible to provide residents with the opportunity to direct their care.

THE POLICY CONTEXT

Although consumer-directed approaches to providing long-term care have gained prominence among policymakers over the past decade, there is much ambivalence toward this concept, particularly with the cash option and other models that allow care recipients to purchase assistance from family and friends. Americans seem more amenable to this concept when it is presented in the form of a tax deduction or tax credit to the care recipient or informal caregiver for services purchased privately. Under the tax incentive approach, an informal caregiver could receive an income tax credit or deduction to offset out-of-pocket expenses for caregiver services. Paid assistance for in-home services, adult day care, and other forms of caregiver respite are supported through current tax plans in a number of states. Those who use such incentives are typically in the middle- or upper-middle-income categories. Such programs seem to be acceptable to the American public, and there are few questions about the appropriateness or quality of consumer-directed services funded in this way.

Greater scrutiny is applied to people receiving services from programs supported by public dollars. When it comes to public programs and dollars, however, there is evidence that the "deserving" (i.e., tax-paying persons who are able to pay for services) and "undeserving" (i.e., those who have come to need publicly funded help of some kind) are treated differently. The guardians of publicly funded long-term care programs, targeted to lower income clients, express serious concern about fraud and abuse, particularly where cash is offered in lieu of a defined service package. In addition, much of the opposition to consumer direction emerges from concerns about the lack of accountability and the inability to adequately protect consumers from physical and emotional harm.

Many Western European countries (e.g., Austria, Germany, and the Netherlands) have included consumer-directed options in their public long-term care programs ranging from caregiver and disability allowances to cash benefits through social insurance (Tilly, Wiener, & Cuellar, 2000). Concerns about fraud and abuse have not emerged as major deterrents to implementation in these societies.

THE EVOLUTION OF CONSUMER DIRECTION

Eustis (2000, p. 10) has noted: "Young adults with physical disabilities, people of all ages with cognitive impairments, and older people with functional impairments share many of the same needs for services and adaptations. However, the professionals and advocates that have traditionally been aligned with each of these groups have different histories and styles of addressing those needs." Whereas consumer direction is currently viewed as applicable to a range of populations, its origins are strongly associated with younger people with disabilities and the desire to control the way in which one receives services and supports. Over the past 40 years, the concept has evolved as it has been explored and embraced, to a greater or lesser extent, by policies and programs targeted to older people with long-term care needs.

The consumer-direction concept initially emerged out of the independent living movement created by college students with physical disabilities in the 1960s and the development of Centers for Independent Living starting in 1972 (Shapiro, 1993). In the 1970s, people with developmental disabilities and mental retardation, including their families and advocates, began to fight for more self-advocacy, culminating in the development of a self-determination movement in the 1980s (Nerney & Shumway, 1996). Advocates of this approach argue that these individuals have the right to direct where, how, and from whom services are provided and to an individual budget to facilitate those choices.

Consumer direction began to be recognized in the aging services and policy communities in the 1980s as advocates for older people and younger people with disabilities found common ground for lobbying purposes (Simon-Rusinowitz, 1999). The Health Care Reform Act of 1993, proposed by the Clinton Administration, included provisions for the development of new home- and community-based care services that offered consumer-directed options to people with disabilities of all ages. The development of assisted living in the 1980s was also based on the premise that older people should have autonomy and choice in their residential and service options and should be empowered to direct their own care. A survey of administrators in state departments of aging, Medicaid, vocational rehabilitation, and mental retardation/developmental disabilities (MR/DD) services indicate that consumer direction options are becoming more available to elderly program beneficiaries in the United States (Velgouse & Dize, 2000). It is important to note, however, that although more than half of all state administrators reported offering consumer-directed programs, MR/DD departments were much more likely than were others to make this option available.

In the mid-1990s, several national initiatives began to create more interest in examining the potential of consumer direction for older as well as younger people with disabilities. The Independent Choices program, sponsored by the Robert Wood Johnson Foundation (RWJF), funded 13 projects (9 demonstrations and 4 research projects) to test new financing and delivery systems that increase consumer choice and direction in home- and community-based services (Velgouse & Dize, 2000). In 1996, the U.S. Department of Health and Human Services and RWJF funded the Cash and Counseling Demonstration to test the viability of offering a cash allowance in lieu of agency-delivered services to people of all ages eligible for Medicaid-covered home/personal programs in Arkansas, Florida, and New Jersey (Mahoney, Simone, & Simon-Rusinowitz, 2000). Preliminary evidence suggests that subsets of older as well as younger people chose consumer direction over a case-managed service package, expressing their preference for controlling their resources and decisions.

STRENGTHS OF CONSUMER DIRECTION

Consumer-directed approaches to long-term care are appealing to people with disabilities because they provide autonomy and choice in decisions about how, where, and by whom services and supports are delivered. Consumer direction affords the client flexibility in how resources are spent, allowing for creativity and the tailoring of services and supports to individual needs and preferences. For working-age people with disabilities, this is seen as essential for maintaining independence in the community. Although a maternalistic attitude toward older people with long-term care needs drove the development of the aging services network over the past 40 years, many elderly people and their families have begun to recognize the advantages of the independence-enhancing, consumer-centered approach that had characterized services for younger people with disabilities. This interest in consumer direction among older people is likely to increase in the future as the baby boomers age and express their preferences for control and choice.

Policymakers are finding consumer direction appealing for several reasons. First, there is the potential for cost savings. Most programs with a cash option, for example, discount the actual amount paid to the clients relative to the cost of a comparable service package. Savings are also realized through the reduction in administrative costs that would have been accrued in managing a service-package program. In addition, resources can be spread further in consumer-directed programs than in conventional, service-package programs. The potential for cost savings is particularly attractive to state officials who currently face serious budget-cutting decisions.

Policymakers are also interested in exploring consumer direction because of the current and projected shortage of home care aides, personal care attendants, and other frontline workers. Consumer-directed approaches afford much more flexibility in hiring workers (including relatives and friends), thus expanding the potential pool of caregivers.

CONSUMER DIRECTION CHALLENGES

There are a number of serious challenges to consumer direction that have impeded the expansion of this approach in the United States.

Cognitive Impairment

Perhaps the most commonly expressed concern relates to consumer direction not being appropriate for all consumers, particularly those with significant cognitive impairment. Advocates for older adults who oppose this approach argue that because the preponderance of elderly people with severe long-term care needs are cognitively impaired, this option would not work for this population. (It is interesting to note that many of these advocates are service providers who are threatened by consumer direction because they see it as usurping some of their market share.)

The literature suggests that consumer direction may be appropriate for certain segments of the cognitively impaired population (Glickman, Stocker, & Caro, 1997; Mahoney, Simon-Rusinowitz, & Simone, 1998). Certainly, elderly individuals who have mild cognitive impairment, or younger people with mental retardation potentially are capable of making decisions about the type of care they want to receive and of having some control over its delivery (Kapp, 2000). For those with severe impairment, family members can work jointly with the individual to direct care decisions, although with the cash option conflict of interest and financial abuse may be a possibility. Nerney and Shumway (1996) argue that support networks or "circles" are crucial to success for many cognitively impaired, developmentally disabled, or mentally retarded individuals. Members of these circles, however, must be freely chosen by, and must have a trusting and respectful relationship with, the person with disabilities.

Some have argued that consumer direction should be seen as specific to certain activities rather than as an "all or nothing" affair (Sabatino, 1996). Consequently, individuals with cognitive impairment may be empowered to control only certain aspects of their care. When their capacity is not adequate, a surrogate decision maker may be necessary. The concept of the surrogate, however, raises a multitude of questions including what characteristics are appropriate for this role, what limits on authority should be imposed, and for consumers without available family members, whether there may be a role for public guardianship in assuming purchasing and oversight decision making (Kapp, 2000).

Potential for Fraud and Abuse

As noted previously, many policymakers are concerned about the potential for fraud and abuse. In addition to concerns about nefarious family members, there is the fear that those receiving the benefits, particularly a cash allowance, will not spend the funds on services or supports related to their long-term care needs. Fraud and abuse are seen as less of a problem where some type of voucher or cash reimbursement is involved, although the potential for "gaming the system" is still viewed as a threat. The Cash and Counseling Demonstration, described in Chapter 3, was designed, in part, to investigate how beneficiaries spend their dollars. It is hoped that the findings will provide new insights into the validity of this concern.

Some opponents of consumer direction do not believe that most people with disabilities, and older adults in particular, have the knowledge and skills to make good service choices. Others are concerned that individuals do not understand what it means to be an employer—to hire and fire workers, to deal with employee benefits such as Social Security and workers' compensation, and to direct one's own care. Consequently, some consumers may misuse the program.

Many public programs wrestling with this concern have devised mechanisms to address this problem (Flanagan & Green, 2000). At least three fiscal intermediary models have emerged in the marketplace over the past decade to assist consumers enrolled in consumer-directed programs with their employer responsibilities. The fiscal conduit, the simplest model, invoices the state for the consumers' grant funds and disburses them to the consumer to manage. The Internal Revenue Service employer agent model and vendor fiscal intermediary models provide a more comprehensive array of fiscal and administrative services including management of employment taxes, and preparation and issuance of payroll checks.

Other support programs have been developed to teach beneficiaries how to be an effective employer and how to direct one's care. These counseling programs, including the one developed for the Cash and Counseling Demonstration, provide training to consumers in such areas as effective hiring and firing practices, purchasing assistive technology and home modifications, and improving communication and conflict resolution skills. The counseling component provides coaching, mentoring, and supportive services to help consumers problem solve and make good decisions about resource use.

Balancing Choice/Autonomy and Safety/Liability

A major concern expressed by skeptics of the consumer-directed approach is how to balance consumer choice and autonomy with safety and protection. A related issue is the question of who assumes liability in consumer direction when something goes wrong—the funder, the client, or the employee? These are particularly thorny issues that have not been, and perhaps will never be, resolved. On the one hand, consumer direction empowers the client to make decisions about how to best use resources to meet one's needs. As long as no health or security problems arise, the consumer and others are generally satisfied. On the other hand, who is responsible for a bad decision? In the litigious United States, the issues of responsibility and liability are particularly volatile and have led many policymakers and public agencies/providers to shy away from consumer direction.

Kapp (2000) identifies a number of issues that need to be addressed in pursuing a consumer-directed approach to long-term care. He notes that the consumer's choices must be predicated on the receipt of adequate information about the foreseeable benefits and risks (informed consent). From a legal perspective, this entails figuring out who has the responsibility to make the information available, identifying the obligations of the consumer to ask the proper questions, and finding remedies for insufficient information sharing. He also underscores the need for mechanisms such as formal negotiated risk agreements to help individuals exercise their prerogative to assume consequences that may be harmful without holding another entity liable (Kapp & Wilson, 1995).

Quality Assurance

One of the major concerns of policymakers is how to ensure and monitor quality in consumer-directed programs. Where agencies are providing defined service packages or contracting out for services, there are ways to establish assessment protocols and measures of accountability that help provide quality oversight. In the consumer-directed approach, the assessment of quality is left primarily to the individual and, if applicable, to their family.

Geron (2000) views the question—can too much choice be a quality problem?—as one of the key "quality riddles" facing policymakers, providers, and consumers. He also identifies another "quality riddle": "Consumers who appear to be satisfied with 'poor' quality care are not poor judges of quality, but rather are using different standards to evaluate their care" (p. 69). He argues that consumers should be left to define quality for the services they know best—nonmedical home care. Consumers must also be involved in the design of satisfaction measures to ensure that the measures fully represent the quality dimensions important to them. Furthermore, consumer-directed programs must meet certain requirements including providing clear information, establishing complaint procedures, and appropriately training consumers and workers.

Potential Worker Exploitation

Some researchers, policymakers, agency-based providers, and unions have raised the concern that consumer direction provides greater opportunity for worker exploitation (Keigher, 1999; Wilner, 2000). It is difficult to monitor the adequacy of wages and benefits, which are already quite low for frontline workers. Studies in Wisconsin and California indicate that independent providers working in publicly subsidized programs tend to have lower wages than those who contract independently on the open market (Cousineau, Regan, & Kokkinis, 2000; Wilner, 2000). In addition, the potential for physical and emotional abuse by clients or their families is greater where individuals have total discretion in hiring and firing home care aides or personal care attendants. As Wilner notes (p. 63): "At its best, consumer-directed care can offer independent providers secure long-term employment with an employer who is dependable, pays on time, and offers consistent hours as well as flexibility in schedules ...At its worst, workers have access to fewer checks and balances, with no external mediator available to either party should difficulties arise".

A number of states have established mechanisms to minimize the potential for worker abuse. As noted earlier, fiscal intermediary organizations not only reduce the burden of being an employer but also ensure that workers get the benefits to which they are entitled. In California, public authorities—quasi-public bodies—have been set up in each county to serve as the "employer of record" for independent home care workers, to engage in collective bargaining for better wages and benefits, and to provide clinical and life skills training. Unions, particularly the Service Employees International Union (SEIU), have successfully organized independent workers in New York and California and have developed special training programs to help home care and personal care aides understand how to work with culturally diverse clients.

Fear of the Woodwork Effect

Many policymakers have expressed their concern that consumer direction, and cash benefits in particular, will encourage people who would otherwise not use services to apply for more flexible benefits. They argue that cash is more appealing than a service package and that consumers would "come out of the woodwork." Studies of programs in other countries (e.g., Germany and Austria) have found no evidence of this outcome; in fact, in the early years of Germany's social insurance program, fewer individuals than expected applied for benefits (Tilly et al., 2000). To minimize the likeliness of a woodwork effect, however, most programs discount the cash benefit relative to the monetary value of a comparable service package. This provides a disincentive for individuals to apply for benefits simply because they want the cash.

CONCLUSION

Consumer direction has emerged as a key policy issue in the area of home- and community-based care. Although the concept began with the independent living, disability rights, and self-determination movements among younger people with disabilities, the approach has gained increased acceptance among many older consumers and advocates for older adults with long-term care needs. Preliminary results from the Cash and Counseling Demonstration in Arkansas, New Jersey, and Florida suggest that when given the choice between cash (a consumer-directed model) and a service package (a more traditional, less consumer-directed managed-care model), many elderly individuals as well as younger people with disabilities choose the consumer-directed option. Most, however, do not want the financial responsibilities of an employer and turn to fiscal intermediaries for assistance.

The future of consumer direction seems promising with the aging of the baby boom generation. More than previous generations of older adults, this cohort is used to making its own decisions and demanding control over how and where services are delivered. Compared to earlier cohorts, a larger proportion of this group of older adults is likely to prefer flexibility in how resources are spent. Younger people with disabilities, furthermore, will be joining the ranks of older adults and will undoubtedly continue their struggle for consumer-directed options. Support for consumer direction, therefore, is likely to grow over the next three decades as the proportion of elderly individuals age 85 and over increases dramatically.

The question remains how policymakers will respond to this demand. If consumer direction is adopted primarily in the form of tax credits for individuals and family caregivers, the benefits will accrue primarily to the more economically advantaged segment of the population. Expansion of consumer direction in publicly funded programs will provide opportunities for lower income older adults who are used to stretching resources and who have demonstrated how to creatively get more with less. These individuals stand to benefit the most from consumer direction if they are free from obsessive oversight driven by fears of fraud and abuse. Although empirical research will shed new light on the potential and pitfalls of this approach, the future of consumer direction in the United States will ultimately be decided on political and ideological grounds.

REFERENCES

Cousineau, M. R., Regan, C., & Kokkinis, A. (2000, February). *A crisis for caregivers: Health insurance out of reach for Los Angeles home care workers.* Report to the California HealthCare Foundation.

Eustis, N. N. (2000). Consumer-directed long-term care services: Evolving perspectives and alliances. *Generations,* Fall, 10–15.

Flanagan, S. A., & Green, P. S. (2000). Fiscal intermediaries: Reducing the burden of consumer-directed support. *Generations,* Fall, 94–97.

Geron, S. M. (2000). The quality of consumer-directed long-term care. *Generations,* Fall, 66–73.

Glickman, L. L., Stocker, K. B., & Caro, F. (1997). Self-direction in home care for older people: A consumer's perspective. *Home Health Care Services Quarterly, 16*(1/2), 41–54.

Kapp, M. B. (2000). Consumer direction in long-term care: A taxonomy of legal issues. *Generations,* Fall, 16–21.

Kapp, M. B., & Wilson, K. B. (1995). Assisted living and negotiated risk: Reconciling protection and autonomy. *Journal of Ethics, Law, and Aging, 1*(1), 5–13.

Keigher, S. M. (1999). The limits of consumer directed care as public policy in an aging society. *Canadian Journal on Aging, 18*(2), 182.

Mahoney, K. J, Simon-Rusinowitz, L., & Simone, K. (1998). Determining consumers' preferences for a cash option: New York telephone survey findings. *American Rehabilitation,* Winter, 24–36.

Mahoney, K. J., Simone, K., & Simon-Rusinowitz, L. (2000). Early lessons from the Cash and Counseling Demonstration. *Generations,* Fall, 41–46.

Nerney, T., & Shumway, D. (1996). *Beyond managed dare: Self-determination for persons with developmental disabilities.* Durham: University of New Hampshire Institute on Disability.

Sabatino, C. P. (1996). Competency: Refining our legal fictions. In M. Smyer, K. W. Schaie, & M. B. Kapp (Eds.), *Older adults' decision-making and the law.* New York: Springer.

Shapiro, J. P. (1993). *No pity.* New York: Random House.

Simon-Rusinowitz, L. (1999, October). *History, principles, and definition of consumer direction: Views from the aging community*. Paper presented at the National Summit on Self-Determination, Consumer Direction and Control. Bethesda, MD.

Stone, R. I. (2000). Consumer direction in long-term care. *Generations*, Fall, 5–9.

Tilly, J., Wiener, J. M., & Cuellar, A. E. (2000). Consumer-directed home- and community-based services programs in five countries: Policy issues for older people and government. *Generations*, Fall, 74–83.

Velgouse, L., & Dize, V. (2000). A review of state initiatives in consumer-directed long-term care. *Generations*, Fall, 28–33.

Wilner, M. A. (2000). Toward a stable and experienced caregiving workforce. *Generations*, Fall, 60–65.

CHAPTER THIRTEEN

Scrutinizing Familial Care in Consumer-Directed Long-Term Care Programs:

Implications for Theory and Research

Chris Wellin

Among the most important and provocative public policy changes affecting long-term care in the United States in recent years is that of consumer-directed care (CDC) (e.g., Benjamin, 2001; Doty, Kasper, & Litvak, 1996; Kunkel, Applebaum, & Nelson, 2003–2004). What distinguishes CDC is an insistence that care recipients' preferences be placed at the model's center. Ascribing decision-making authority to people who have traditionally been seen as passive (if grateful) objects of medical/professional control involves a fundamental shift in perspective, for researchers and practitioners alike (Yamada, 2001).

In this chapter, I reflect, in a constructively critical way, on the burgeoning literature on CDC for older adults. My analysis is informed by a *critical gerontology* perspective (e.g., Estes & Linkins, 2000; Holstein & Minkler, 2003; Luborsky & Sankar, 1996). My focus is on the implications of *familial* caregiving within CDC programs, which has proven to be a significant precondition for their expansion as a policy option. Despite the centrality of familial care to the expansion of CDC, the extensive literature on this approach has not fully explored its implications. Despite the culturally and politically normative aura surrounding familial care, we need to address the question, as Strawbridge and Wallhagen did (1992): whether "all in the family is always best."

I discuss four interrelated themes that are important for understanding and assessing CDC in the future: (1) structural labor problems in paid caregiving, (2) the tendency to idealize familial caregiving compared to paid care in the public sphere, (3) neglect of class and gender stratification in the provision of care work, and (4) distortions contained in the market metaphor in which consumer-directed care is embedded.

SITUATING AND REFLECTING ON CDC RESEARCH

In principle, everyone advocates wider discretion for disabled people regarding the nature and scheduling of care. However, questions regarding who specifically provides care, and the extent to which programs and policies such as CDC address the broader public policy context and supports surrounding familial care warrant more attention. A large body of prior theory and research strongly suggests that, without fundamental improvements in the provision of *extra-familial* care, in the public sphere, demands placed on familial caregiving will intensify, even as demographic trends reveal the inadequacy of this model as a long-term solution to challenges of societal aging. Furthermore, overreliance on familial care will inevitably exacerbate class and gender inequity and divert attention from structural reforms in the caring labor force which are central to overarching policy goals (see Strawbridge & Wallhagen 1992). I agree with Keigher (1999, p. 206), who writes, "The key public policy question should be how well [CDC] arrangements serve all sectors of communities in need, including the providers of care." Meeting this goal will require critical reflection on select implications of CDC—for familial and non-kin caregivers alike. The latter group has not been a central focus of the literature on CDC. However, my experiences as a paid caregiver[1] and a sociologist of work and occupations have sensitized me to issues of non-kin care. In turn, my assessment of the literature on CDC is less sanguine than is typical of authors in this volume.

Most prior research on CDC—by evaluation researchers and advocates of community-based care options for older adults—has been strongly positive about its benefits for those with chronic disabilities (e.g.,

---

[1] In the late 1980s, I worked for some 18 months as a paid caregiver in a residential care facility for older adults with cognitive illnesses; I followed this experience with nearly 2 years of ethnographic research in this setting, including observation and interviews with paid staff and residents' family members (see Wellin & Jaffe, 2004).

Doty, 2004; Eckert, San Antonio, & Siegel, 2001; Keigher, 1999; Yamada, 2001). To achieve greater control and flexibility in both the manner and scheduling of their care, care recipients or "consumers" in such programs are permitted to act as employers, ostensibly free to hire and fire caregivers. Though hiring familial caregivers is but one among a wider set of options available to participants, in fact doing so has proven to be the most common arrangement.[2] This finding is the point of departure for my argument. As employers, consumers are able to channel public funds (e.g., through Medicaid waivers granted to states or local tax levy programs) to care providers, an arrangement designed to shift control from agency personnel to care recipients. CDC clients have, in fact, been shown to perceive greater control, autonomy, flexibility, and satisfaction in daily care arrangements than has generally been true either in institutional care or in conventional agency-governed programs employing home health aides. Care recipients, policy advocates, and academics alike celebrate these findings.

What is equally clear is that CDC programs, in various forms, are here to stay. As Benjamin (2001) points out, several conditions have converged to reinforce this policy agenda: effective advocacy by disabled adults of all ages, consumer movements challenging the dominance of medical personnel and controls, concerns over dramatic increases in the demands and costs of long-term care, the Supreme Court's recent "Olmstead" decision mandating "least restrictive" community care options for the disabled,[3] and a serious shortage of direct care workers—all have contributed to the momentum among governmental policymakers and private foundations to advance and assess CDC initiatives. Also, CDC models resonate with prevailing political realities and cultural norms in the United States: these include, respectively, the contraction and devolution of welfare state policies and filial (read *women's*) obligations to assume, to the extent possible, responsibility for elder care.

In the past decade or so, the CDC model has expanded beyond its historical connections with younger disabled persons and has been implemented and evaluated in programs serving older adults. But as this model becomes more firmly established, it is essential that researchers and

---

[2] I use the term familial to refer to family members and friends, with whom recipients may enjoy kin-like relations (see Bould, 1993.)

[3] Passed on 1999, the Supreme Court's Olmstead decision mandates that "states are required to place persons with ... disabilities in community settings rather than in institutions when the State's treatment professionals have determined that community placement is appropriate, the transfer from institutional care to a less restrictive setting is not opposed by the affected individual, and the placement can be reasonably accommodated, taking into account the resources available to the State and the needs of others with ... disabilities."

advocates for long-term care options examine CDC from various theoretical and substantive angles. Yamada (2001) is helpful in clarifying our
need to consider implications of CDC for particular groups of *stakeholders*: these include care recipients, familial and other caregivers, professionals such as social workers who are central in coordinating agency-
based care, government/policy actors, and even researchers. Inevitably
there are tradeoffs in social policies, regarding costs and benefits for particular groups. Thus an important part of the future agenda for CDC
researchers will be to examine such tradeoffs, in an attempt to reconcile tensions and better integrate the model in the overall system of long-
term care.

Taking a step in this direction, in this chapter I develop several areas
of critique (listed later) that address the origins, limitations, and even the
language/discourse of CDC in prior literature.[4] My central focus is the
impact of CDC on family caregivers, with an eye toward issues of gender
equity and the larger context of public support for caregiving. In addition to developing several themes that, in my view, invite caution in our
adoption of CDC, I address underlying problems regarding its relation to
efforts that address enduring structural problems in paid caregiving. My
argument is that CDC and efforts to enhance the system of non-familial
care are best seen as *complementary, rather than competing*, policy
agendas.

APPLYING A CRITICAL GERONTOLOGY PERSPECTIVE

My analysis is informed by the *critical gerontology perspective* (e.g., Estes
& Linkins, 2000; Holstein & Minkler, 2004; Luborsky & Sankar, 1996).
This approach proceeds from concrete research topics and terminology
in our field—which, as with CDC, are often specialized and technical—
and opens them up to reflective scrutiny. Critical gerontology utilizes such
established theoretical perspectives as political economy and feminist theory, "whose standpoints can unsettle familiar and conventional ways of
thinking by revealing their often-unrecognized underlying values and consequences" (Holstein & Minkler, 2004, p. 788). Luborsky & Sankar
(1996, pp. 99–100) write that, having defined and contextualized—
whether culturally or historically—a particular topic, the goal of critical
gerontology is to reveal . . . gaps and limitations in the concept/problem

---

[4] We should reflect carefully on the connotations and implications of terminology in public
policy discourse; as Lakoff and Johnson (1980, pp. 10–13) argue, metaphors have the power
either to "highlight or hide" important dimensions of public issues. In concluding the chapter
I return to a discussion of the uses and problems of this metaphor for CDC research.

formulation's ability to explain the phenomena it focuses on, and other problems it does not highlight."

A critical gerontology approach, then, aims not to refute, but to extend or reframe questions and findings in a topical area, better to inform research and practice. Fraser and Gordon (1997, p. 619) are correct in writing that "such a critique is not merely negative. By questioning the terms in which social problems are named, we expand the collective capacity to imagine solutions." By emphasizing what I see as problematic issues in CDC, I hope to sharpen that "imagination" and to use CDC as a strategic site to consider issues of general relevance to social research on aging, family, and caregiving.

As a policy initiative affecting the lives of extremely vulnerable people, and given the inadequacies and indignities of institutionally based long-term care, CDC provokes strong reactions; this applies to researchers and policy analysts, as well as to clients, their friends and family members, and occupational groups such as case managers, for whom the implications of CDC are complex and far-reaching. Equally important is the magnitude of the public–private partnership that has coalesced around CDC: the National Council on Aging, the U.S. Department of Health and Human Services, the Robert Wood Johnson Foundation, and the Centers for Medicare and Medicaid Services, academic research institutes in several states—all have invested financial and staff resources in support of CDC pilot programs and their evaluation. All of these groups, along with the policymakers and government entities involved in CDC, are stakeholders with distinctive interests and perspectives on the policy. As such, they have commitments that inevitably shape how they define CDC—both as a public policy and as an object of social research.

Like any analyst, my view of CDC is similarly filtered through particular disciplinary and topical concerns. Jaffe and Miller (1994) point out that the social experiences, interests, and concepts we bring to studying a particular problem create *positionality*—distinct angles of vision that shape how we assess research questions and answers. This argument echoes Becker's important earlier (1970) essay, "Whose Side Are We On?" His point was partly that there are *always* value positions in our research, and that we should strive to make them—and the scope of our inquiry—clear, and thus less apt to cloud or distort the inferences we make. He argues further that charges of bias are especially likely if/when our research challenges "hierarchies of credibility" (p. 126) by advocating for groups that have been marginal or discredited. Ironically, CDC researchers' strong and legitimate identification with care recipients may obscure the broader web of ties and consequences affecting those on whom "consumers" depend for expanded care options.

CDC, DISABILITY, AND CHALLENGES OF LATE LIFE

A review by Ungerson (2000) shows that CDC is but one among a spectrum of policies—many in Western Europe and the UK—that since the 1970s have allowed public cash allowances to support familial caregiving. She argues that, over time, the primary goals and constituencies of such policies have changed: an early focus in the 1970s on addressing the poverty that often accompanies disability, shifted in the 1980s to efforts to compensate the value and gendered nature of caring work. More recently, in the 1990s, advocacy for CDC has centered on disabled people's entitlement to dignity, autonomy, and control over the care they receive. This current framing of the policy in the United States has de-emphasized problems of poverty and gender equity (Hess, 1985); issues of familial norms and obligations in CDC, if raised at all, have generally been portrayed as benign (i.e., as conditions that stimulate and enhance the quality of care). Contractions in welfare state policies and fiscal constraints, though implicit, are simply assumed in current policy and academic discourse.

In the United States, the roots of CDC can be traced to the Independent Living Movement (ILM) of the 1960s and 1970s, which was driven by demands by younger disabled adults for maximal autonomy in their everyday lives (Benjamin & Matthias, 2001; Eustis, 2000). In contrast, many CDC pilot programs currently being carried out and evaluated across the United States involve disabled *older* adults, including those with multiple chronic conditions and even cognitive illnesses such as Alzheimer's disease. Such conditions, and the dependence they engender, are difficult to square with assumptions about autonomy and self-determination that are central to the philosophy and administration of CDC.[5] Understanding better the implications of life-course differences is important in how we conceptualize and administer CDC programs. Although the ILM aimed to achieve autonomy for disabled adults both *in* the community and *from* their family networks, CDC for elders has proved to be highly dependent on family care. Given the qualms—both cultural and personal—many elders have, about "being a burden" to one's children, and the intensification of work demands facing men and women alike in the United States, this is a provocative finding. Whether elders' preference for kin care is a product of general assumptions about filial obligation, particular care demands, negative prior experience with paid care, or of a tendency to concentrate one's circle of intimate others in late life (see Carstensen, 1995) are empirical questions that deserve careful attention from researchers.

---

[5] See Collopy (1988) for an important conceptual taxonomy of autonomy.

Furthermore, there are major differences in health status and in the *trajectory* of disability among groups at different stages of the life course. The health status of younger disabled adults, for example, those who are employed but wheelchair bound, is often fairly stable. Typically it is characterized by a "plateau" of functional adaptation in which maintenance of independence at home is a basis for pursuing goals in education, work, and recreation (Benjamin, 2001, p. 86). In contrast, health trajectories of older adults are more likely to be volatile or even progressive. A fruitful theme in the future research agenda regarding this care model will be to explore, theoretically and empirically, the extent to which and how life-stage and life-course dynamics (e.g., the nature and quality of social roles and relations that are salient for the disabled person) shape the experience and optimal administration of CDC programs.[6]

From the standpoint of social service administration, CDC challenges the traditionally hierarchical, professionally dominated *medical model* in aging services (e.g., Morgan & Kunkel, 2001, pp. 346–349; see Conrad 1987). Inadequate fiscal, regulatory, and evaluation constraints have also hampered the quality of care, including that provided in the community through the "home health" industry (Applebaum & Phillips, 1990; Estes & Close, 1998). Thus, implementing CDC has required personnel such as case managers and social workers to alter their role and mission, along with the regulatory constraints they have regarded as protective of client safety and quality of care. In the past it was assumed (e.g., Benjamin, 2001) that the CDC model was limited in its relevance for older adults because of the demands it imposes on clients to manage employment relations, paperwork, and complicated third-party payment procedures. Also, health and social services for older adults have traditionally been more subject to formal case management and regulatory rules than have those involving younger adults. Such rules, and the web of professional practices that support them, were a major barrier to early CDC pilot programs enacted as part of Medicaid's home and community-based services. Currently, arrangements such as allowing for "authorized representatives" to oversee fiscal management have helped in overcoming these barriers, which in turn has allowed for expanded enrollment.

Research on CDC confirms, however, that the traditional system of rigid standards has not only proved to be inadequate to assure high-quality care and client control but also "[tended] to limit or inhibit client and family caregiver involvement in such critical areas as hiring and firing

---

[6] Moreover, prior research by Jaffe (1989) on intergenerational home sharing suggests that the perceived success and duration of dyads depends in good part on the extent to which dyad members' respective goals and capacity for independence are in synch.

decisions and the scheduling and day-to-day supervision of aides" (Doty et al., 1996, p. 402). It is clear, then, that participation in CDC is driven not only by attractive "pull" factors (including greater flexibility and freedom in choosing care providers and schedules) but also by factors that "push" people away from agency-based care or that have limited the availability such care. What is important to consider is that complaints about the quality of care that are often targeted at agency-based *providers* could as appropriately be directed at the *regulatory constraints* under which aides have worked. Persuasive research (e.g., Aronson & Neysmith, 1996: Eustis & Fisher, 1991; Karner, 1998; Piercy, 2000) reveals that care recipients and paid providers (no less than family care providers) share many priorities and preferences regarding the meanings of, and conditions necessary for, excellent care. Still, when combined with the poor labor conditions facing paid caregivers, which chronically undermine the quality and continuity of care, these regulatory strictures have placed severe limits on the ability of clients to negotiate and sustain satisfying lives despite disability.

Historically, reluctance to extend CDC and other innovative programs to disabled older people has also reflected deeper cultural barriers. Cohen (1988, p. 25) calls attention to what he terms the "Elderly Mystique," an implicit, paternalistic form of ageism which assumes "that when disability arrives, hope about continued growth, self-realization, and full participation in family and society must be abandoned so that all energy can be directed to avoiding the ultimate defeat, which is not death, but institutionalization, which is regarded as a living death." These cultural biases compound the regulatory and occupational constraints on the autonomy of older adults with disabilities. So it is not surprising that CDC researchers have concentrated on such constraints, more than they have on broader issues and implications surrounding the policy.

Established Foci of Applied Research on CDC

Research on CDC has thus far emphasized applied, policy-relevant questions, such as how we might best plan, implement, and evaluate consumer-directed care programs. Inasmuch as such programs operate currently in more than half the states in the United States, the importance of generating and disseminating evaluation research is clear.

At the conference in 2001, which was a forum for several of the chapters in this book, and generally in the policy literature, CDC has been examined through the prism of professional, administrative, and analytic/research questions. Among them are the following. How are the roles of conventional agency personnel such as case managers likely to change in CDC programs, and how can we overcome occupational barriers to its implementation? When and how should we incorporate CDC programs into long-term care planning? What kind of information is essential for assessing the appropriateness of particular enrollees for participation in CDC? How should we revise our quality indicators for CDC to include consumer perspectives? How can we translate such data on quality into program administration? Can we document significant improvements in consumers' satisfaction with care, in CDC versus agency-based arrangements? As my co-authors in this book attest, answers to these questions have important and wide-ranging implications, particularly for stakeholders directly involved in administering or evaluating CDC programs. But, broader scrutiny of this policy calls for a mode of analysis that extends such questions and connects them with related streams of research.

POINTS OF DEPARTURE FOR CRITICAL INQUIRY INTO CDC

Having sketched the larger context of my interest, I explore several of the key assumptions and questions that have been central in researchers' discourse on CDC in recent years. I believe there has been too narrow a focus regarding some questions, and the omission of others, that are central to sociological theory and research in carework. Four interrelated problems I address are:

1. Structural employment/labor problems that afflict paid caregivers and care recipients;
2. A tendency to idealize (in effect if not by intent) familial caregiving in contrast to paid care in the public sphere;
3. Class and gender inequity in the provision of care work, which CDC seems potentially to exploit and to reproduce;
4. Distortions contained in the market metaphor in which consumer-directed care is embedded.

Structural Work Problems That Afflict Paid Caregivers and Care Recipients

The emergence of CDC as a policy option has been driven partly by a looming crisis in the recruitment and retention of paid care workers. This problem has been long in the making; it reflects such large-scale economic and policy conditions as inadequate insurance reimbursement and limits on levels of third-party payments as well as on limited personal resources of elders needing home care (Kane, 1989). More recently, Noelker (2005) and Atchley (1996) are among those who have shown that the pool and stability of the caregiving workforce is woefully inadequate to meet the needs of an aging society. Atchley (p. 18) reports: "This shortage is projected to reach crisis proportions very soon. Indeed, chronic short-staffing of nursing homes and waiting lists stemming from a shortage of home care workers are a reality in many areas already." Roots of this shortage are laid bare in the U.S. Department of Labor Statistics *Occupational Outlook Handbook*. For example, it is clear to anyone who has had a hospital stay or cared for a family member that such work requires sensitivity and skill. Yet in the labor market, "Personal and Home Care Aides" are defined and compensated according to an instrumental and demeaning image of what constitutes caring work. The *Handbook* reports that:

> [Such aides] help elderly, disabled, and ill persons live in their own homes or in residential facilities instead of in a health facility. Most work with elderly or disabled clients who need more extensive care than family members or friends can provide . . . They clean clients' houses, do laundry, and change bed linens. Aides may plan meals . . . shop for food, and cook. Aides also may help clients move from bed, bathe, dress, and groom. Some accompany clients outside the home, serving as a guide and companion.

The report goes on to report an optimistic job outlook for such workers, who numbered more than 400,000 in the year 2000, because of unusually high employment growth in this sector—especially for those entering elder care. On the other hand, we read that recruitment is undermined because "Turnover is high, a reflection of the relatively low skill requirements, low pay, and high emotional demands of the work" (http://www.bls.gov/oco/ocos173.htm).

As of the year 2000, the median hourly earnings of personal and home care aides was $7.50 per hour/$1,200 per month (with visiting home health aides earning a dollar less, and those in residential care facilities somewhat more). More recently (2005), the Service Employees International Union reported that nearly one-fifth of direct care workers they represent, who are single parents, qualify to receive Food Stamps. As Atchley (1996) points out, the problems of low pay are compounded by an absence of health insurance and other employee benefits (which are especially inadequate for *independent* care providers, such as most in CDC) and by an absence of mechanisms that promote continuity of care and other sources of job satisfaction. He concludes, in fact, that "major predictors of job satisfaction include continuous orientation programs that give aides a collective voice and sense of belonging in the employing organization; ongoing training to extend and refine skills in caregiving; and shared decision-making and flexible supervision to address employees various needs" (p. 18; and see Wilner, 2000). Unfortunately, few employers furnish these benefits, and so chronic problems of turnover and lack of public trust in paid care persist.

This pattern is sadly ironic, in that several researchers (e.g., Aronson & Neysmith, 1996; Foner, 1994; Wellin & Jaffe, 2004) have documented paid caregivers' strong commitment to those for whom they care, and their resourcefulness in circumventing bureaucratic and other barriers to humane caring relationships (see also Eustis & Fisher 1991; Stone, 2000a). Cancian (2000) reviewed research in a range of care settings— including hospitals and nursing homes—with an eye to the provision of paid *emotional care*. In bureaucratic settings, which tend to fragment caring relations into instrumental tasks, such care tends to be invisible or even discouraged; it is rarely acknowledged or compensated as part of the work routine. Yet Cancian (2000, p. 148), too, finds this to be a salient theme among paid caregivers and concludes that "The quality of emotional care...depends in large part on specific characteristics of the organization in which the caregiver works." There is ample evidence, then, that the quality and continuity of paid elder care are influenced by structural work conditions and incentives that have repeatedly been found to operate in occupations that many regard as more "professional" than caregiving.

Although the vast majority—roughly 80%—of care continues to be provided by informal sources (friends and family), the need for a more extensive and better system of public/paid care becomes more urgently apparent over time. As Bengston et al. (2003) show, this is truly a global phenomenon. Falling death and birth rates portend that, in the future, fewer children and extended family members will be available to care for a growing proportion of people over the age of 65 in the United States (Wallace & Estes, 1996). Noelker (2005, p. 2) reports that, by the year 2030, we will see a 6% decrease in the U.S. population ages 18 to 64 and a 27% *increase* in the population ages 85 and over. Her analysis indicates that, "The ratio of potential informal caregivers (family and friends) will decrease by some 40% between now and the year 2030." In addition, decades of research has confirmed that the quality of familial relationships, between disabled people and care providers, is enhanced when the latter are relieved of some of the burden of giving daily instrumental care (e.g., Bowers, 1990; Smith & Bengston, 1979). There is equally wide consensus that, rather than shirk caregiving tasks, informal care workers assume as much of this responsibility as is possible for them.

A large body of evidence leads inescapably to the implication that future policy should ideally support improvements in the quality and stability of paid caregiving (in the private and public sectors), as an essential condition for disabled people and their families. However, although the extensive literature on CDC has in passing noted the labor crisis in paid care as a condition for the emergence of CDC, rarely has it addressed whether or how this policy helps to address the root causes of that crisis. In the absence of any explicit analysis of what underlies the shortage of staffing, trust, and continuity in paid care arrangements, research celebrating CDC can have the effect of "blaming the victims" (here, paid caregivers) for exploitative labor market conditions and, in turn, creating an invidious comparison between familial and public care provision. To the extent this is true, a potential implication of research on CDC may be a tendency to idealize (in effect if not by intent) family caregiving in contrast to care in the public sphere.[7] My argument is that these *structural* conditions in paid carework must be addressed, irrespective of who provides care and, furthermore, that failure to address such conditions will only increase reliance on kin care.

Ideals and Limitations of Familial Caregiving

The focus of my critique is the prominent role *familial* caregiving plays in existing CDC programs. This pattern is hardly surprising, inasmuch as family members continue to provide the great majority of such care for elders generally. A note on terminology: in the chapter title, I refer to *familial care.* I use this term, rather than "family care," for empirical and conceptual clarity: first, care recipients in CDC programs are generally permitted to pay either relatives (defined by blood or marriage ties), or friends; second, it has long been recognized (e.g., Stack, 1974) that the term *family* often describes informal, reciprocal networks of emotional and material support based on extended as well as "fictive" kinship (Bould, 1993). It is especially understandable that the commitment of poorer people—as most CDC clients are, as indicated by their eligibility for Medicaid—to familial obligations may take precedence over the conventional "rationality" of individual self-interest. Thus, in practical terms one's ability to take advantage of CDC is typically dependent on existing networks of familial support. This reality is hard to reconcile with the more atomistic market/consumer metaphor.

A recent study, based on a nationally representative sample, found that over 90% of community-dwelling elders get some unpaid help from family, and some two-thirds of them rely exclusively on family supports. Doty (2004, p. 3) reports that they receive a weekly average of 75 hours of assistance, of which 60 are estimated to come from family members. Thus,

---

[7] Obscuring dynamics of care, and the perspective of the disabled person, in family discourse is distorting, just as Conrad (1987) and others argued was true of the imposition of medical categories on illness experience.

despite the growing need for elder care—and the conflicting demands of work and child care that challenge family caregivers—we continue to provide it largely through private, voluntary efforts. But what of the compelling need for *extra-familial* support?

It is important to point out, then, that CDC programs contain two related but separable components: the first is an increase in the *types and amount of control* the care recipient is granted, regarding the scheduling and provision of care tasks. (In principle, such control can also be exerted over agency-based care providers and would indeed seem to be most necessary in that case, given that agency-employed workers have limited knowledge of care recipient's needs and lack the filial obligation required naturally to adapt care tasks.) The second component in most CDC programs is *expanded freedom to recruit and hire* care providers (termed "workers" by administrative personnel, as opposed to the "consumer" who receives care). The pool of eligible caregivers is expanded in CDC to include not only home-health agencies or freelance care workers, but also one's network of family members and friends. It is conceptually and also empirically important not to conflate these two issues, because consequential dynamics of caregiving, and of the relationships shared by particular care providers and receivers, vary independently.

We have the benefit of many sensitive studies of home care, some focusing on family caregiving (e.g., Abel, 1990; Corbin & Strauss, 1988; Kosberg, 1992), others on professional/paid home care workers (e.g., Karner, 1998; Piercy, 2000; Piercy & Dunkley, 2004; Rivas, 2003). This research offers remarkable consensus in terms of the expressed ideals and criteria, among all concerned, regarding high-quality care: it requires a sensitive blending of instrumental and socioemotional care, with respect, warmth, and a desire to adapt to individual needs and preferences (Wellin & Jaffe, 2004). What is understandably less well studied and understood, however, is the *integration* of paid and familial caregiving, through the auspices of social policy initiatives such as CDC.

Issues of familial care provision have been a recurring, if not a salient, theme in the growing literature on CDC. Others have noted this trend (e.g., Brown & Foster, 2000; Feinberg & Whitlatch 1998; Kunkel et al., 2003–2004), but none to my knowledge has made it the center of attention. Although informal/family support has historically met most elder care needs, increases in women's labor force participation and the general intensification of work hours and demands in the United States are compounding demographic pressures of societal aging that strain family resources (Bengston et al., 2003). Further, the social bases and implications of this reliance on familial support, in a culture that so prizes independence (from family and institutional constraints alike), deserves careful scrutiny

(Strawbridge & Wallhagen, 1992). Also problematic is the stubborn pattern of gender inequality in the distribution of caregiving responsibility. It continues to be true, as Brody (2004) and others document, that women are often *caught in the middle* of conflicting role demands—as workers, carers, and community/volunteer actors. Abel (1990), examining the phenomenon of daughters caring for aging parents, found that the emotional and practical demands of family care can be overwhelming, even in economic circumstances that are more stable and less stressful than is likely to be true for many CDC participants. Pearlin and colleagues (e.g., Pearlin, Pioli, & McLaughlin, 2001) provide a stream of research that persuasively shows that role disruptions, rooted in long-term care demands, has a negative impact on care workers' health status. In turn, a body of earlier research (e.g., Pillemer & Wolf, 1986) warned against and documented the risks of *elder abuse*, as a result of demands placed on family caregivers, and of declining health status among family caregivers, caught between conflicting role demands (Pearlin et al.) or simply subject to *role fatigue* (Goldstein, Regnery, & Wellin, 1981). Necessary gains for disabled adults, of whatever age, should not impose a prohibitive cost for care providers—including those who, as friends or family members, are normatively expected to fulfill this role.

Context and Tradeoffs of Familial Care in CDC

As stated, research has shown that extending CDC to elder care has relied heavily on the involvement of family and friends, both as care providers and as proxies or "authorized representatives" helping to arrange and monitor payment for care. Although clients have the option to hire friends, family members, or independent aides (e.g., though classified ads), a clear majority—from 60% to 80%, depending on the program under review—has in fact chosen to hire those whom they know. The author of a recent review of the *Cash and Counseling* Program (operating in Arkansas, New Jersey, and Florida) reports, further, "the preference for hiring family members was strongest among elders" (Doty, 2004, p. 6). This finding begs the empirical question of whether the CDC option injects a modest cash reward into preexisting familial care arrangements or, on the other hand, provides an incentive that activates new caring relations and arrangements. It is safe in any case to conclude, first, that the viability of consumer-directed care for older adults, especially those with severe physical or cognitive impairments, will depend significantly on the participation of family members; and second, that this participation inevitably imposes tradeoffs for family caregivers regarding how they allocate time, energy, and resources between compelling and competing obligations (Kapp, this volume). A fuller understanding of the impact of these tradeoffs, and of their consequences for CDC and for larger debates in long-term care policy, requires that researchers contextualize this initiative in the current political/policy environment, and also that we integrate the growing body of CDC research findings with relevant streams of prior research. Among the most relevant are those dealing with caregiver stress/burden, labor conditions and politics in the service economy, family dynamics, and gender inequality.

Class and Gender Inequality in the Provision of Carework

Beyond demographic constraints are fundamental issues of social justice and equality that require improvement in the cultural and economic value we place on caring work (Stone, 2000b). As Glenn (2000, p. 89) argues, "keeping the family as the 'natural' unit for caring relationships helps anchor the gender division of caring labor . . . and disguises the material relationships of dependence that undergird the arrangement." This points up another troubling silence, in public advocacy and CDC research, regarding class and gender inequalities. These inequalities shape the lives of participants in myriad ways. Whether they are Medicaid eligible, or become involved through various community-based care programs, participants in CDC are both poor and beset with chronic and/or progressive disabilities. Middle-class and affluent families are increasingly reliant on "subcontracting" care responsibilities for children and for disabled members; they are able to exert substantial control over care arrangements, and to obtain high-quality, reliable care by virtue of their ability to pay (see Hochschild, 2002, pp. 185–223, *passim*). For the poor, the sheer lack of disposable income is but one of a larger set of cumulative disadvantages, which are manifested in old age and shape the normative and practical negotiation of familial care.

In this connection, De-Ortiz (1993) analyzed New York City's Medicaid-funded home attendant program, via the political economy perspective. She argues that "the elderly poor's health conditions, and thus their need for care, must be examined within the context of their labor histories and the poverty they have confronted and endured throughout their lives . . . The cumulative effects of poverty, including nutritional deficiency, inadequate housing, and lack of medical care, also affect the health of the elderly and their need for care" (p. 24). She goes on to point out that substandard housing, not to mention such neighborhood factors as safety and access to basic goods and transportation—all contribute to health status and to the ability of people to access and mobilize resources they need to remain independent.

How is this point connected to the operation of CDC? It is axiomatic in the literature in gerontology that one's ability to remain at home and avoid institutionalization is shaped by support networks as much as by health status per se (e.g., Gubrium & Sankar, 1990). Clients' heavy reliance in CDC programs on familial care reflects long-standing relations of reciprocity and extended kin networks most strongly characteristic of poorer people. Middle-class and affluent families stress "human capital" investments and assume autonomy in pursuit of greater earning potential. Poorer workers, however, are often mired in the service or informal economies and thus have more tenuous and more episodic involvement in wage work. Under such conditions, family members are more likely to stay in geographic proximity with one another, and more accustomed to accommodating daily life to the exigencies of survival among the larger group. It is easy (and too common) to romanticize the resilience of such extended family forms, but they often impose serious constraints and "opportunity costs" on members who, in contrast to middle-class norms may see family more as a community of fate (than of choice). To the extent this is true, CDC is a policy that may respond to the needs and preferences of older disabled people, at the cost of longer term quality of life and income security among younger care providers. To the extent this is true, family care is a significant mechanism for the transmission of intergenerational poverty. Of course, it is an empirical question whether and how caregivers are able to balance their demands under CDC with those of work outside the home, however there is suggestive evidence (i.e., a finding that caregivers provide an average of some 8 hours of care per day) that doing so is challenging.

So far, we have said little about the gender dynamics of child care and elder care, so unchanging have the patterns remained (e.g., Brody, 2004; Calasanti & Slevin, 2001, pp. 146–152). Both at home and in the paid caregiving workforce, the predominance of women is taken for granted (excepting male home health aides responsible for handling immobile clients). The recent gains among women in the labor force and professions, and the success of so many as single parents, depend on their ability to afford or share care responsibilities in ways that preserve their viability as wage or salaried workers. Any caregiving policy that rests on women's work in the home—even if modestly paid—is a threat to this progress. Thus, although the rhetoric and research that is supportive of CDC celebrates the *empowerment* of the recipient/consumer, from a feminist angle it may rather appear as a *re-privatization* of care in the home, in line with an ideology of fiscal austerity, and on the shoulders of the very women who are at the highest risk of facing poverty and ill health in their own later years. More, CDC can be seen to be consistent with a larger trend of policy devolution (from the federal to state and local governments) as noted by Estes and Linkins (2000, pp. 160–162).[8] The importance of ensuring quality of life for care recipients should not obscure attention to macro-level conditions underlying the emergence and ultimate role of CDC as a policy option. To sum up, I have argued that both the demand for and development of CDC have rested on a largely implicit basis of class inequality. Buttressing kin-care via CDC will not by itself either relieve or exacerbate these deeply entrenched patterns. However, there is a potential danger that policy incentives that draw more poor women into kin-care will compound their disadvantage in terms of education and employment, even as it enhances life for those for whom they care. An implication of this argument is that those seeking to expand CDC should, as Stone (2000b) urges, make common cause with related movements to address structural problems in the social status and rewards for care in the workforce,[9] and that theoretical analyses and evaluations of CDC programs need to recognize and address class and gender processes which (through the mechanism of familial care norms) the policy may exploit and reinforce.

Potential Distortions in the Consumer/Market Metaphor

A final critical theme concerns the conceits and potential distortions of the "consumer/market" metaphor with which policy makers and researchers define and discuss CDC. As cultural critic Raymond Williams and others (Best, 1995; Lakoff & Johnson, 1980) have shown, metaphors have social consequences; they shape how we think about and act toward contested social problems. Metaphors are central to how we *typify* social problems, that is, how we categorize and treat them. As Best (p. 9) explains, particular typifications "emphasize some aspects and not others, they promote specific orientations, and they focus on particular causes and advocate particular solutions." As such, the language we use to represent social problems can limit how we perceive their scope, as well as our realm of power to affect them through policy intervention. It should be apparent, based on the discussion thus far, that the consumer/market metaphor is problematic when applied to care decisions in CDC.

Strictly speaking, a *consumer* is defined as an autonomous individual who acquires a product or service in a competitive market. In a founding

---

[8] Indeed, a condition of introducing one CDC pilot in Ohio was that it be "revenue neutral"—cost no more than existing programs.

[9] These coalitions must include the growing union movement among care-workers and others in the allied health professions. Delp and Quan (2002) offer an important analysis of how unionization was part of a successful grass-roots strategy to enhance the working conditions and rewards of home care workers in California.

document of cultural studies, *Keywords,* Williams (1976, p. 69 emphasis, in original) notes that the "decline of *customer* used from the 15th century on to describe a buyer or purchaser is significant, in that *customer* had always implied some degree of regular and continuing relationship to a supplier, whereas *consumer* indicates a more abstract figure in a more abstract market." Whereas market transactions are generally impersonal and ephemeral, family ties of reciprocity are embedded in dense emotional and material bonds, stretching across long periods of time (Groger, 1992).

For all these reasons, the consumer/market metaphor seems strained at best when applied to severely disabled people whose only other options are nursing home residency or reliance on agency-employed health aides. The term is further strained when considering the prevalence of familial care in CDC: both the decision to enter into CDC and the negotiation over care within dyads is profoundly determined by the resources, traditions, and sentimental order of family life (including extended or fictive kin). The desire, however deeply felt, to promote or maximize dignity and self-determination among the disabled should not thereby create blindness to powerful conditions of their lives and social networks.

Conceptually, the agency of *consumers* is derived from a premise, not of entitlement or material equity, but rather of metaphorical freedom in a market. Robyn Stone (2000, p. 6) suggests that it is important to distinguish between *consumer choice* and *consumer direction*: "With . . . managed care and Medicare (at least in theory) offering a range of plans as well as a fee for service option, the elderly and younger disabled are facing more choices in how they receive their healthcare. . . . Consumer direction, however, focuses specifically on the degree to which people are proactive in making decisions about care, including the hiring and firing of workers and the oversight of services." For most CDC clients, whose limited resources qualify them for Medicaid funding, the range of choices is quite narrow. For them CDC offers choice in the confined but important domain of how and from whom they get care. However, the choice is constrained in the public sphere by virtue of the shortage and instability of "frontline" staff support, and so for most this choice, and the control it aims to gain, can only be exercised in practical terms when family or friends are both available and willing to take part.

So, how well does the consumer metaphor capture these realities of interdependence? In many ways the image of the consumer—of an isolated and autonomous actor in a market—hides as much as it reveals about the social relationships that underlie CDC. The image has the rhetorical and pragmatic virtue of resonating with a larger policy environment that, since the Reagan years, has stressed contraction of the federal welfare state and privatization in the realm of health and social services (Wallace

& Estes, 1996). For advocates of this connotation of consumer control (a group which I am *not* implying includes CDC researchers), the symbolic freedom to take risks and benefits in the marketplace (as in the ongoing debates about the private accounts in Social Security, or of "local control" in economically strapped urban schools [Lewis & Nakagawa, 1995] takes precedence over the traditional paternalism of formal regulation. This faith in markets tends to elide, when it does not oppose, the universalistic and redistributive aims of welfare policies and the recognition of class/gender inequality. Nonetheless, this image of consumerism tends, in effect, to isolate the care recipient from their supportive, familial network, recasting relations of interdependence into quasi-employment relations. A material expression of this shift is that, in CDC, the care recipient is designated as both employer and client, ostensibly free to hire and fire care providers. Recasting the disabled person, from a subject of formal and bodily regulation to an active agent directing their care, has both symbolic and practical power. Indeed, this shift is central to claims for why CDC is *empowering* for care recipients.

Nonetheless, I conclude with references to insights that help to convey the potential dangers of distorted metaphors in the present case. First, Riger (1993, p. 279) develops a conceptual critique of *empowerment*. She concludes that, although valuable, the term is suffused with assumptions and values of individualism, "leading potentially to unmitigated competition and conflict among those who are empowered; and . . . a preference for traditionally masculine concepts of mastery, power, and control, over traditionally feminine concerns of communion and cooperation." So, empowerment is problematic not only because it can lead us to focus narrowly and to obscure relational and contextual dynamics (in this case, bearing on caregiving), but also because it can promote—even among familial networks—zero sum competition which may strain the already delicate fabric of families coping with hard times. The other caveat, in closing, I take from the social theorist Ralf Dahrendorf. Analyzing the nature of "life chances" (1979, p. 31), he argues that they are determined by a combination of *options and ligatures* (or, said differently, choices and enabling social ties). These he says can be in an "optimal relation" with one another: "A maximum of options is not by itself a maximum of life chances, nor is a minimum of options the only minimum of life chances. Ligatures without options are oppressive, whereas options without bonds are meaningless." In the transition from pre-modern societies, Dahrendorf argues, one's fate was largely determined by ligatures, by social ties; we enjoyed few choices that were independent of our ascribed community. In light of our investigation of CDC, and of the prominence in such programs of family care provision, one rightly wonders whether the rhetoric of *consumer choice* might obscure a realization of the continued (and now formally sanctioned and compensated) role of family ties in the future of elder care for less affluent families in the United States.

CONCLUDING REMARKS

I have been struck by the passionate support of CDC by care recipients and scholars. During a conference on CDC several years ago, I attended a panel discussion involving participants who are currently enrolled in CDC programs in Ohio. One could not but be moved by the testimony of people for whom involvement in CDC has allowed greater control and dignity in everyday life, despite serious and chronic illness. According to Cohen (2004), these progressive goals define, or should, what we mean today by quality in long-term care. My earlier work and research in residential care (Wellin & Jaffe, 2002, 2004) has taught me how disabilities can become defining features of interaction and identity for older people, even for those fortunate to live in comparatively privileged material conditions. From this standpoint, placing care recipients at the center of research and policy is a progressive, even radical, shift, and one that is a necessary though not sufficient condition for reform (also see Conrad, 1987).

Any incremental change in long-term care policy, such as CDC, faces a daunting test: it must reconcile legal, ethical, and cost issues, and also seek to preserve the flexibility and humanity of caring relations. As difficult as these challenges are currently, they also entail longer range issues of generational and gender equity (Hess, 1985). Societal aging, combined with low fertility rates and intensifying work demands for women and men, is exposing a pervasive set of problems that have plagued paid caregivers and the quality of paid care; these include the cultural and economic devaluation of paid care work, chronic instability, and turnover in paid care relations, and racial/ethnic and class divisions between care providers and care recipients (Glenn, 1992). We know empirically (e.g., Benjamin, 2001, p. 82; Feinberg & Whitlatch, 1998) that, regardless of age, disabled people share many priorities regarding the care they receive: they value safety, continuity, flexibility, and sensitivity to individual needs and preferences. These qualities are, of course, neither necessarily present in family ties nor absent in paid/agency-based care. But so long as the structural problems of paid caregiving remain unresolved, public distrust will continue and familial care will represent not only a historical norm but also a misguided cultural ideal. Demographic change, however, in conjunction with the "social imperative" to consider the needs and rights of major groups of stakeholders, requires that we address broader problems in the labor market and service economy.

Some readers may think it far-fetched or alarmist to connect CDC with these broader problems. However, CDC presents a prominent focus of current policy attention and, as such, deserves wide-ranging scrutiny from gerontologists and others with a commitment to addressing long-term care needs. While the public spotlight shines, we need to reveal the broader nature of the caregiving challenge. The weight of my critique in this chapter has been skeptical, but not negative, regarding the findings and implications of prior research on CDC. My questions, and the implications I draw, extend those of others, and my concerns about the wider context of CDC in no way diminish those of others who have studied the policy from other vantage points.

In fact, my critical stance cannot resolve profound dilemmas that have arisen with respect to caregiving research and public policy. One of these concerns a contradiction between my position here and other analyses of the use of public dollars to support *child care*. Many researchers (e.g., Oliker, 2000) who share my premises and policy goals decried the end of Aid to Families with Dependent Children (AFDC) and the imposition of work mandates for single mothers instituted as part of the Clinton Administration's welfare "reform." A central point raised by such writers was that it is wrong to deny funding to poor women who choose to devote their energies to caregiving (as we celebrate among more affluent mothers), especially given what has proven to be the limited options that await them as wage workers. More broadly, Schwartz (2002) makes a compelling case that the historical tendency in the United States for federal and state policies to provide lower levels of funding to kin (than non-kin) caregivers reflects a societal devaluation of caring. In seeking to resolve this contradiction, one could argue that parents choose to have children, as adult children cannot choose to have disabled parents; similarly, one could argue that adults' general preference for independence and autonomy should temper our emphasis on any social policy that might infringe on it (for adults of whatever age). However, these positions betray an ad hoc quality, which only underscores the cultural and political complexity of the issues involved. With respect to CDC, I have argued *not* that we remove this as a policy option, rather that for many reasons it should not be the *only* or default option available to disabled older adults and their families.

In the end, all social policies contain and touch multiple realities; each is important and is shaped by contextual factors that make reconciling them all the more difficult. My goal has been to develop lines of inquiry that will reinforce the centrality of CDC in several related areas of theorizing and research in the social sciences. I have explored questions which I feel are crucial to address in the future, but which have been either implicit or tangential in the growing body of applied research in this area.

In the near future, I look forward to adding to empirical knowledge of CDC in my own research, and to the lively debate and clarification that I have tried to promote.

ACKNOWLEDGMENTS

I am grateful for guidance and suggestions of Robert Applebaum, Suzanne Kunkel, and Matt Nelson. Sally Bould, Christine Caffrey, Elias Cohen, Carroll Estes, Glenn Muschert, Edward Wellin, and the editors provided helpful comments on earlier drafts. An earlier version of this paper was presented at the 4th Annual Conference of the Carework Network, San Francisco, California, in August 2004.

REFERENCES

Abel, E. K. (1990). Daughters caring for elderly parents. In J. F. Gubrium & A. Sankar (Eds.), *The home care experience* (pp. 189–208). Newbury Park, CA: Sage.

Applebaum, R., & Phillips, P. (1990). Assuring the quality of in-home long-term care: The 'other' challenge for long-term care. *The Gerontologist, 30*(4), 444–450.

Aronson, J., &. Neysmith, S. M. (1996, February). You're not just in there to do the work: Depersonalizing policies and the exploitation of home care workers' labor. *Gender & Society*, 10(1), 59–77.

Atchley, R. C. (1996). Frontline workers in long-term care: Recruitment, retention, and turnover issues in an era of rapid growth. *Ohio Long-Term Care Report, Scripps Gerontology Center,* Miami University, Oxford, OH.

Becker, H. S. (1970). Whose side are we on? In *Sociological Work* (pp. 123–124). New Brunswick, NJ: Transaction.

Bengston, V. L., Lowenstein, A., Putney, N. M., & Gans, D. (2003). Global aging and the challenge to families. In V. L. Bengston & A. Lowenstein (Eds.), *Global aging and challenges to families* (pp. 1–24). New York: Aldine De Gruyter.

Benjamin, A. E. (2001). Consumer-directed services at home: A new model for persons with disabilities. *Health Affairs, 20*(6), 80–95.

Benjamin, A. E., & Matthias, R. E. (2001). Age, consumer direction, and outcomes of supportive services at home. *The Gerontologist, 41*(5), 632–642.

Best, J. (Ed.). (1995). *Images of issues* (2nd ed.). Hawthorne, NY: Aldine De Gruyter.

Bould, S. (1993, March). Familial caretaking: A middle-range definition of family in the context of social policy. *Journal of Family Issues, 14*(1), 133–151.

Bowers, B. (1990). Family perceptions of care in a nursing home. In E. K. Abel & M. K. Nelson (Eds.), *Circles of care* (pp. 278–289). Albany: SUNY Press.

Brody, E. M. (2004). *Women in the middle: Their parent years* (2nd ed.). New York: Springer.

Brown, R., & Foster, L. (2000). Cash and counseling: Early experiences in Arkansas. *Issue Brief: Mathematica Policy Research, Inc.*, (1), 1–2.

Calasanti, T. M., & Slevin, K. F. (2001). *Gender, social inequalities, and aging.* Walnut Creek, CA: Alta Mira Press.

Cancian, F. M. (2000). "Paid emotional care." In M. H. Meyer (Ed.), *Care Work: Gender, labor, and the welfare state* (pp. 136–148). NY: Routledge.

Carstensen, L. L. (1995). Evidence for a life-span theory of socioemotional selectivity. *Current directions in psychological science, 4*(5), 151–156.

Cohen, E. S. (1988). The elderly mystique: Constraints on the autonomy of the elderly with disabilities. *The Gerontologist, 28*(Suppl.), 24–31.

Cohen, E. S. (2004). Milestones in the quest for quality. *The Gerontologist, 44*(1), 127–133.

Collopy, B. J. (1988). Autonomy in long term care: Some crucial distinctions. *The Gerontologist, 28*(Suppl.), 10–17.

Conrad, P. (1987). The experience of illness: Recent and new directions. In J. A. Roth & P. Conrad (Eds.), *Research in the sociology of health care* (Vol. 6, pp. 1–32). Greenwich, CT: JAI Press.

Corbin, J., & Strauss, A. (1988). *Unending work and care.* San Francisco: Josey Bass.

Dahrendorf, R. (1979). *Life chances.* Chicago: University of Chicago Press.

Delp, L., & Quan, K. (2002, Spring). Homecare worker organizing in California: An analysis of a successful strategy. *Labor Studies Journal, 27*(1), 1–23.

De-Ortiz, C. M. (1993). The politics of home care for the elderly poor: New York City's medicaid-funded home attendant program. *Medical Anthropology Quarterly, 7*(1), 4–29.

Doty, P. (2004). Consumer-directed home care: Effects on family caregivers. *Policy brief* from the National Caregiver Alliance, National Center on Caregiving.

Doty, P., Kasper, J., & Litvak, S. (1996). Consumer directed models of personal care: Lessons from Medicaid. *The Millbank Quarterly, 74*(3), 377–409.

Eckert, J. K., San Antonio, P. M., & Siegel, L. (2001). The cash and counseling qualitative study: Stories from the independent choices program in Arkansas. University of Maryland Center on Aging.

Estes, C. L., & Close, L. (1998). Organization of health and social services for the frail elderly. In S. M. Allen and V. Mor (Eds.), *Living in the community with disability* (pp. 73–94). New York: Springer.

Estes, C. L., & Linkins, K. W. (2000). Critical perspectives on health and aging. In G. Albrecht et al. (Eds.), *Critical perspectives on health and aging* (pp. 154–171). London: Sage.

Eustis, N. N. (2000). Consumer directed long-term care services: Evolving perspectives and alliances. *Generations, 24*(3), 10–15.

Eustis, N. N., & Fischer, L. R. (1991). Relationships between home care clients and their workers: Implications for quality of care. *The Gerontologist, 31*(4), 447–456.

Feinberg, L. F., & Whitlatch, C. J. (1998). Family caregivers and in-home respite options: The consumer-directed versus agency-based experience. *Journal of Gerontological Social Work, 30*(3/4), 9–28.

Foner, N. (1994). *The caregiving dilemma.* Berkeley: University of California Press.

Fraser, N., & Gordon, L. (1997). Dependency demystified: Inscriptions of power in a keyword of the welfare state. In R. E. Goodin & P. Pettit (Eds.), *Contemporary political philosophy: An anthology* (pp. 618–633). Oxford, UK: Blackwell.

Glenn, E. N. (2000). Creating a caring society. *Contemporary Sociology, 29*(1), 84–94.

Glenn, E. N. (1992). From servitude to service work: Historical continuities in the racial division of paid reproductive work. *Signs, 18*(1), 43.

Goldstein, V., Regnery, G., & Wellin, E. (1981, January). Caretaker role fatigue. *Nursing Outlook, 29*(1), 24–30.

Groger, L. (1992). Tied to each other through ties to the land: Informal support of back elders in a southern U.S. community. *Journal of Cross-Cultural Gerontology, 7,* 205–220.

Gubrium, J. F., & Sankar, A. (1990). *The home care experience.* Newbury Park, CA: Sage.

Hess, B. (1985). Aging policies and old women: The hidden agenda. In A. S. Rossi (Ed.), *Gender and the life course* (pp. 319–332). Hawthorne, NY: Aldine DeGruyter.

Hochschild, A. (2002). *The commercialization of intimate life.* Berkeley: University of California Press.

Holstein, M. B., & Minkler, M. (2003, December). Self, society, and "the new gerontology." *The Gerontologist, 43*(6), 787–796.

Jaffe, D. J. (1989). *Caring strangers: The sociology of intergenerational home-sharing.* Greenwich, CT: JAI Press.

Jaffe, D. J., & Miller, E. M. (1994). Problematizing meaning. In J. F. Gubrium & A. Sankar (Eds.), *Qualitative methods in aging research* (pp. 51–66). Thousand Oaks, CA: Sage.

Kane, N. M. (1989). The home care crisis of the nineties. *The Gerontologist, 29*(1), 24–31.

Karner, T. X. (1998). Professional caring: Homecare workers as fictive kin. *Journal of Aging Studies, 12*(1), 69–82.

Keigher, S. M. (1999). The limits of consumer-directed care as public policy in an aging society. *Canadian Journal on Aging,* 18 (2), 182–210.

Kosberg, J. I. (Ed.) (1992). *Family care of the elderly.* Newbury Park, CA: SAGE.

Kunkel, S. R., Applebaum, R. A., & Nelson, I. M. (2003–2004). For love and money: Paying family caregivers. *Generations* (Winter): 74–80.

Lakoff, G., & Johnson, M. (1980). *Metaphors we live by.* Chicago: University of Chicago Press.

Lewis, D. A., & Nakagawa, K. (1995). *Race and educational reform in the American metropolis.* Albany: SUNY Press.

Luborsky, M. R., & Sankar, A. (1996). Extending the critical gerontology perspective: Cultural dimensions. In J. Quadagno & D. Street (Eds.), *Aging for the twenty-first century* (pp. 96–103). New York: St. Martins.

Morgan, L., & Kunkel, S. (2001). *Aging: The social context* (2nd Ed.). Thousand Oaks, CA: Pine Forge.

Noelker, L. S. (2005). Strengthening the long-term care workforce: Avoiding the pending crisis. Keynote Lecture to the Annual Meeting of the Ohio Association For Gerontology in Education, Aurora, OH.

Oliker, S. J. (2000). Examining care at welfare's end. In M. H. Meyer (Ed.), *Carework: Gender, labor, and the welfare state* (pp. 167–185). New York: Routledge.

Pearlin, L. I., Pioli, M. F., & McLaughlin, A. E. (2001). Caregiving by adult children: Involvement, role disruption, and health. In R. H. Binstock & L. K. George (Eds.), *Handbook of aging and the social sciences* (5th ed., pp. 238–254) San Diego, CA: Academic Press.

Piercy, K. W. & Dunkley, G. J. (2004, September). What quality care means to family caregivers. *Journal of Applied Gerontology, 23*(3), 175–192.

Piercy, K. W. (2000, August). When it is more than a job: Close relationships between home health aides and older clients. *Journal of Aging and Health, 12*(3), 362–387.

Pillemer, K. A., & Wolf, R. S. (Eds.). (1986). *Elder abuse: Conflict in the family.* Dover, MA: Auburn House.

Riger, S. (1993). What's wrong with empowerment? *American Journal of Community Psychology, 21*(3), 279–292.

Rivas, L. M. (2003). Invisible labors: Caring for the independent person. In A. R. Hochschild & B. Ehrenreich (Eds.), *Global woman* (pp. 70–84). New York: Metropolitan Books.

Schwartz, A. E. (2002, September). Societal value and the funding of kinship care. *Social Service Review,* 430–459.

Service Employees International Union. (2005). Expanding the workforce: a key ingredient to cash and counseling. Web newsletter of July 29, 2005; *www.SEIU.org.*

Smith, K. F., & Bengston, V. L. (1979). Positive consequences of institutionalization: Solidarity between elderly parents and their middle-aged children. *The Gerontologist, 19*(5), 438–447.

Stack, C. B. (1974). *All our kin.* New York: Harper Torchbooks.

Stone, D. (2000a). "Caring by the book." In M. H. Meyer (Ed.), *Carework: Gender, labor, and the welfare state* (pp. 89–11). NY: Routledge.

Stone, D. (2000b). Why we need a care movement. *The Nation,* March 13, 2000.

Stone, R. I. (2000, Fall). Introduction to consumer direction in long-term care. *Generations, 24*(3), 5–9.

Strawbridge, W. J., & Wallhagen, M. I. (1992). Is all in the family always best? *Journal of Aging Studies, 6*(1), 81–92.

Ungerson, C. (2000). Cash in care. In M. H. Meyer (Ed.) *Carework: Gender, labor, and the welfare state* (pp. 68–88). New York: Routledge.

U.S. Department of Labor Statistics. (2006–2007) Occupational outlook handbook, *2006–07* edition (Bulletin 2600). Washington, DC: U.S. Government Printing Office. (*http://www.bls.gov/oco/ocos173.htm*).

Wallace, S. P., & Estes, C. L. (1996). Health policy for the elderly. In J. Quadagno & D. Street (Eds.), *Aging for the twenty-first century* (pp. 483–498). New York: St. Martins.

Wellin, C., & Jaffe, D. J. (2002). Clock time versus story time: Temporal and narrative dimensions of care for the fragile self. Working paper, Center for Working Families, University of California, Berkeley.

Wellin, C., & Jaffe, D. J. (2004, August). In search of personal care: Barriers to identity support for cognitively impaired elders in residential facilities. *Journal of Aging Studies, 18*(3), 275–295.

Williams, R. (1976). *Keywords: A vocabulary of culture and society.* Glasgow: Fontana.

Wilner, M. A. (2000). Toward a stable and experienced caregiving workforce. *Generations, 24*(3), 60–65.

Yamada, Y. (2001). Consumer direction in community-based long-term care: Implications for different stakeholders. *Journal of Gerontological Social Work, 35*(3), 83–97.

CHAPTER FOURTEEN

Gifts or Poison?
The Cultural Context of
Using Public Funds to Pay
Family Caregivers

Lisa Groger

"To give is to show one's superiority."

—Marcel Mauss, *The Gift*

From time to time, analysts from the United States and from less-developed countries raise the question of whether they might learn something about health care policy and related matters from European democracies. These "model" countries have long traditions of supporting social policies and programs designed for the purpose of shoring up the economic security of families. Often this question of learning from other countries is rhetorical. When it is posed more seriously, analysts invariably come to the conclusion that whatever those other countries do might not work here. And they are probably right, because health care and elder care policies are deeply embedded in specific cultural contexts and, therefore, cannot be adopted easily and piecemeal into cultural contexts with different values and belief systems.

The existence of cash allowances to families who care for elders, or the lack of such support, illustrates to what extent the larger cultural context shapes not only the outcome of the policy processes but also the ethical questions and moral concerns about this particular phenomenon. Concerns about the effects of paying family caregivers for doing what they are "supposed to do anyway" include the fear that such payments might taint a supposedly altruistic relationship or lead to abuse or low quality of care; or that such arrangements might exploit the labor of low-income women for tasks no one else is willing to do and thus marginalize these women even more by keeping them out of the "real" labor force. This chapter draws on the work of others to describe types of cash payments currently available to family caregivers in several Western European countries. The conditions that appear to foster the policies and practices of compensating family caregivers in these selected countries is described, and whether and to what extent similar conditions exist in the United States is examined. I argue that the existence, impact, and perception of various forms of direct or indirect payments to family caregivers cannot be fully understood unless they are examined within their cultural contexts.

All industrialized nations recognize, and acknowledge through social policies, that family caregivers to dependent and disabled relatives need financial assistance. Each country demonstrates this recognition to a greater or lesser degree than others. Non-industrialized nations are becoming increasingly concerned about how to value and support informal care, as witnessed by the list of 59 countries that paid long-term care cash allowances in 1987. The list of these developing countries includes, but is not limited to, Algeria, Benin, Bolivia, Chad, China, Libya, Togo, and Zaire. Developed countries that recognize this need for financial support include, but are not limited to, France, Sweden, Germany, Spain, Italy, Greece, Switzerland, Great Britain, the Netherlands, and Norway (Linsk, Keigher, Simon-Rusinowith, & England, 1992, p. 41). All of these countries have social insurance systems. Many support family caregiving either through "constant attendance allowances" or through supplemental payments to family caregivers who look after old or disabled relatives. These kinds of payment are discussed next.

Some countries compensate caregivers under either the disability or the work injury provision of their social security act. Countries employ a variety of ways in which to compensate family caregivers. Some do so in the form of hourly wages; others provide various forms of reimbursement on a fee-for-service basis; yet other governments pay direct allowances to family members who provide personal care, chore service, homemaker services, and the like, to an elderly relative (Linsk et al., 1992, p. 21). Lastly, a number of countries offer a tax credit or tax deduction as incentive for providing informal care. For example, Canada has several types of means-tested tax benefits for caregivers; Germany provides tax benefits to family caregivers regardless of income; and Japan provides minimal tax credit to workers who care for frail elders. In the United States, the Dependent Care Tax Credit is means-tested and limited to caregivers who provide at least 50% of the care and reside with the care recipient (Montgomery & Feinberg, 2003).

TYPES OF CASH PAYMENTS TO FAMILIES

All European and most other Western industrialized countries have one or several of the three major types of cash disability allowances for long-term care (LTC): constant attendance allowances, family allowances, and invalid care allowances.

According to Linsk and colleagues (1992) constant attendance allowances are "cash payments to individuals who need assistance with activities of daily living, household tasks or personal care, or supervision. They permit mentally competent beneficiaries to use their limited cash grant to design a package of goods and services which they feel maximizes the reduction in personal discomfort with which they are encumbered by their disability" (Linsk et al., 1992, p. 50). Constant attendance allowances provide a supplement to regular benefits payable either under the disability or retirement provisions of their social insurance systems. The benefit amount is usually calculated either as a percentage of the disability pension or as a percentage of a worker's previous average earnings, or paid as a flat rate or amount. Some countries index the amount of this supplement to the cost of living. Attendance allowances add between 20% and 100% to pensions, bringing total benefits to between 85% and 125% of previous average wage earnings (Linsk et al., pp. 52–53).

Some analysts see a direct relationship between the creation and the growth of constant attendance cash allowances in the form of cash and two historical events. The first event was World War II and the resulting shortage of caregivers, which was alleviated through cash payments that disabled elders could use to hire professional or family labor. The second event was the emergence of national universal health care systems, which allowed a streamlining of eligibility determination. Now, in many countries, a family physician, rather than several layers of bureaucrats, determines entitlement based on national guidelines (Linsk et al., 1992, p. 51). Current payments to caregivers must be seen in the larger historical and social context of countries with a long-standing and well-established philosophy about the role of the state in the well-being of individuals. For countries in which health and education are considered a universal birthright, the inclusion of LTC is a logical step when dictated by the aging of a society. In such a context it is much easier to solve the problem of caregiver shortage by paying family caregivers and trusting elders to manage their care provision.

Family allowances paid for each child are the second type of benefit that must be considered as part of the context in which to evaluate cash payments for elder care. It is usually paid as an allowance per child to all families, regardless of need, with the amount increasing for each subsequent child. In most European countries, family allowances were instituted not only to encourage procreation but also to redistribute resources and to combat poverty. Although not explicitly intended for elder care, family allowances, together with other direct or indirect benefits, nevertheless help all families with children, thus protecting and supporting members who are also caregivers to elders.

The third type of cash payment to families is invalid care allowances. These payments resemble family allowances in the broadest sense, providing special social protection for non-employed caregivers directly or indirectly. They can operate as allowances under the branches of social security (e.g., old age and invalidity, sickness, or work injury), as part of protection for spouses, or as compensation directly for loss of time from occupational employment (Linsk et al., 1992, pp. 50–51).

There are considerable variations both between and within countries in the amounts of cash allowances paid to caregivers, but even the smallest amounts must be seen within the context of the total service system of which they are a part, and which include universal health care, the role of unions in shaping benefits, universal family allowances, and the definition of the role of the state in individual welfare.

For example, in 1994, Germany passed the Long-Term Care Insurance Law as a fifth pillar of the Social Security system. The four other pillars are health, unemployment and accident insurance, and old-age pension, all of which are mandatory and universal (Reichert & Naegele, 1999). Long-term care insurance is financed through a 1.7% tax on gross salary or wages equally shared by employers and employees. In the case of pensioners, the premiums are paid by a pension insurance fund. Employers resisted this new law but negotiated a means of transferring some of the cost to consumers by abolishing one of Germany's public holidays. Employees had to give up the equivalent of 1 day's paid holiday. This does not seem an exorbitant price to pay, given that in Germany, every worker starts with a basic minimum of 1 month of paid vacation, in addition to at least a half dozen religious holidays sprinkled throughout the year. Thus the universal and compulsory nature of long-term care insurance makes it affordable by spreading both financing and risk across the whole population. Eligibility is based solely on health care needs as assessed by professionals. No means testing is involved, thus no stigma is attached to receiving long-term care services paid for by government money. Germany's long-term care insurance offered several innovations:

- Persons in need of care who are entitled to benefits can choose between in-kind and cash benefits. Clients who choose cash payments are then able to pay a family member or any other person they may choose to hire.
- Long-term care insurance pays contributions to the pension fund of the caregiver in case he or she is not otherwise employed, or is employed fewer than 30 hours a week as long as the caregiver provides care for at least 14 hours a week. In other words, long-term care insurance contributes to both the current and the future financial security of the caregiver.
- Long-term care insurance has led to an expansion of a variety of in-home services, which indirectly support family caregivers. These include day- or night-care service; caregiver respite through short-term (up to 4 weeks) institutional care for the care recipient; funds for modifying homes for persons with disabilities; and funds for personal care articles such as diapers, special soaps and creams, and appliances such as hospital beds, wheelchairs, walkers, toilet chairs, as well as prosthetic devices.

In considering the drawbacks or downside of this policy, German analysts Reichert and Naegele (1999) note that the first two innovations mentioned previously might act as incentives for paid caregivers to give up work. By doing so, they would lose, without realizing it, some employment-related factors such as social support from, and contact with, co-workers, which are seen as potential buffers against the stress associated with caregiving. The authors refer explicitly to the loss of the respite function of the workplace (p. 36) and postulate that this loss might have a negative influence on the caregiver/care recipient relationship. They also fear that middle-aged women may find it difficult to re-enter the labor force after their caregiver job is over. It seems to me that these concerns are quite different from those expressed in the United States, where some analysts worry about how the infusion of money might taint the caregiver/care receiver relationship. The suggestion here is that the questions we ask must also be seen in the larger sociopolitical and policy contexts in which they arise.

SIX COUNTRIES COMPARED TO THE UNITED STATES

Viola Lechner and Margaret Neal's (1999) edited volume on *Work and Caring for the Elderly: International Perspectives* provides information about 11 countries: Canada, Germany, Great Britain, Israel, Japan, Sweden, the United States, Brazil, Mexico, China, and Uganda. In this chapter the comparison is limited to the 11 most developed of these countries because of the similarities of their institutional structures and their longer standing history of producing the economic surplus required for the emergence of the welfare state. The developing countries discussed by Lechner and Neal face different challenges, making them less appropriate models for possible emulation by the United States.

Lechner and Neal (1999, p. 223) conclude that "exemplary programs are universal, affordable [long-term care] services for elders and universal paid temporary work leaves for employed caregivers." They suggest that three interrelated conditions contribute to the development of such supports: (1) external pressure, (2) ability, and (3) willingness.

External Pressure

This is exemplified by demographic trends typical of aging societies. These trends include women's increasing labor force participation, smaller birth cohorts supplying fewer caregivers for growing numbers of elders in need of care, and the resulting conflict between work and caregiving obligations of those who provide care.

Ability

Countries must have the requisite economic and social infrastructures both to afford and to administer a comprehensive system to effectively respond to their growing demands for care.

Willingness

External pressures and ability to respond in terms of resources are strikingly similar in all seven developed countries discussed by Lechner and Neal (1999). However, these countries vary widely in their willingness to provide comprehensive supports for employed caregivers and their elders. The countries with the strongest, most comprehensive support, or the highest degree of willingness, share the following characteristics: (1) strong unions that aggressively buttress the interests of all workers by obtaining concessions from both government and employers; (2) centralized governments that foster universal systems and that avoid the fragmentation of policies, programs, and practices inherent in systems that delegate legislative and other powers to multiple levels; (3) universal health care which provides a conceptual and practical framework for adding new services; and (4) less-developed private sector initiatives due to a pervasive and dominant role of the state in social welfare matters.

Based on the aforementioned conditions and criteria, Sweden ranks highest in terms of unionization of its work force, centralization of government, extent of its universal health care system, and general role of the government in economic affairs. In contrast, the United States ranks lowest on these same criteria, and the other five countries (Canada, Germany, Great Britain, Israel, and Japan) fall between these two extremes. Specifically, in Sweden, 90% of the workforce is unionized; Sweden's government is characterized by strong central planning, an extensive public welfare system, and a relatively small private sector. Israel ranks similarly to Sweden with regard to a highly unionized labor force, though its private sector is slightly more developed than Sweden's and is slightly less developed than that of the United States. Germany, Great Britain, and Canada each have a labor force that is 33% unionized, a private sector that is less developed than that in the United States, and strong public support. For example, eligibility for Germany's long-term care services is universal and based on health care needs, whereas similar services in Canada and Great Britain are means-tested. In Japan, 25% of the labor force is unionized; the government engages in highly centralized planning and close working relationships with business, and it has a universal long-term care program (Lechner & Neal, pp. 227–228). In contrast to the aforementioned countries, in the United States only 15% of employees are unionized; it has highly decentralized political power and institutions, and, according to Lechner and Neal, "Its reliance on coalition building makes it very difficult for government, even if it wanted to, to develop coherent economic and social policies that would lead to the initiation of LTC services for all, paid family leaves, and other family focused benefits. Moreover, the private sector is much more developed in the United States than in other developed countries, especially in the areas of LTC services and supports for employed caregivers" (p. 228). Thus, institutional/structural arrangements together with their attendant cultural traditions provide a climate in which universal public support of family caregivers may either find fertile ground or not be able to take root. Table 14.1 summarizes the differences and similarities in these seven countries.

According to surveys conducted in 1985 and 1990 by Linsk and colleagues (1992), 35 states in the United States had programs in place that paid some compensation to family caregivers of elders. Although there are great variations in how these decentralized programs are structured, none of the programs conceives of payments to family caregivers

Table 14.1 Summary of Comparison

	Sweden	Israel	Germany	Great Britain	Canada	Japan	United States
Percentage of workforce unionized	90%	90%	33%	33%	33%	25%	15%
Centralized governments	Yes	Yes	Yes	Yes	Yes	Yes	No
Universal health care	Yes	Yes	Yes	Yes	Yes	Yes	No
Relative role of private sector	Small	Medium	Medium	Medium	Medium	Medium	Large

as a universal entitlement. Instead of being provided under such universal programs as Social Security, family allowances in the United States are always means-tested and largely financed by Medicaid waivers. In other words, only poor people qualify for these services after having demonstrated that they are both poor and deserving. One could argue that the stigma associated with such welfare programs greatly limits their potential effectiveness for easing the burden of family caregivers on any measurable scale. Linsk and colleagues show in great detail how these programs in the United States are driven by considerations of cost effectiveness. To quote from their 1992 study: "The extent to which cost effectiveness (saving state money) dominates all discussion of home care services today appears to corrupt rather than facilitate rational consideration of family caregiver compensation schemes. In fact, the cost effectiveness of community care remains unknown" (p. 93). Unknown or not, the argument of cost effectiveness makes perfect sense within the larger U.S. sociocultural/ideological context and public discourse which proclaims the virtues of limited government and individual responsibility. Within this framework, it also makes perfect sense to consider economic success and good health as the result of either personal initiative or shortcoming. The explanatory power of structural forces that beget poverty is completely ignored in this discourse. The power to make things happen, good or bad, resides in individuals. Within this ideological context of individual responsibility and self-reliance, it is easy to argue that public moneys would contaminate the sacred sphere of the family. Or so the story goes. It all makes perfect sense, in spite of the growing burden U.S. families face because of an increasingly aging population, just as it makes sense for German, French, and Swedish families to look to the government for their basic safety net.

In other Western democracies, constant care allowances are driven by recognition of the social value of caring for elders at home. Compared to the United States, European countries have made a greater commitment of resources to attendance allowances, and this is clearly reflected in the fact that the United States devotes the lowest percentage of gross national product to Social Security. It is important to note that in most other industrialized countries, Social Security is much more broadly defined than in the United States and includes not only universal health insurance but also an array of other direct or indirect payments that benefit families generally and caregivers to elders specifically.

In their thoughtful policy recommendations, Linsk and colleagues (1992) present several alternative approaches to allocating money for payments to family caregivers in the United States, and they examine these for their ability to accommodate prevailing political and cultural core values. Although the authors are favorable to reconsidering an approach based on the recognition that caregiving in itself is a value, they conclude that a deficiency framework using means-testing, quite elaborate bureaucracies, and quite rigid mechanisms of monitoring would have a better chance of being adopted in the United States. In other words, the politically feasible solution to this problem would also be culturally appropriate by using the structures and involving stakeholders already in place. The army of professionals in the service of elders—the "Aging Enterprise"—itself is the product of the perception of elders as helpless, not only in need of services but also in need of paternalistic guidance provided by professionals, who happen to thrive financially under this arrangement. The only culturally and politically compatible solution to the caregiving problems of the United States is one that would not present a threat to the Aging Enterprise.

To conclude with two, more or less testable, hypotheses:

1. The less money a government is willing to allocate for paying family caregivers, the more vociferous the expression of concern that cash payments to caregivers will undermine the moral fabric of the family.

   The study by Linsk and colleagues (1992) found that in the United States, bureaucrats were the only "stakeholders" who expressed this concern. The beneficiaries of cash payments expressed satisfaction with the arrangement. Payment validated the care family members were providing, and it enabled elders to reciprocate for the care they were receiving. Far from tainting their relationship, the injection of money helped to keep it solid and equitable by empowering both parties.

2. The more embedded cash payments to family caregivers are in the larger system of social welfare, the easier it is to make such allocations.

The European social democracies have a long history of supporting families. For example, both France and Germany have long-standing traditions of paying family allowances for each child from birth to age 18, starting with a relatively small amount for the first child and increasing amounts for subsequent children, regardless of need. The clear intention of these payments was to motivate couples to have more children, and to reward them for raising children. In my own research in France in the mid-1970s among family farmers, such family allowances could account for the equivalent of the income of a family farmer (Groger, 1984). In Germany, a woman who has worked outside the home and who is vested in the national pension system received a pension supplement for each child she raised. The step from such family allowances for raising children to allowances for caring for elders is a logical one in such a context. In Germany, universal health care was the vehicle onto which universal long-term care insurance was hitched, and paying family members for long-term care services is an equally logical step, particularly when it costs much less than would institutionalization. Whether and to what extent cash allowances to families actually enable families to buy services readily and in sufficient quantity and quality is another question, one that must be explored at the micro-level of the consumer (Jani-Le Bris, 1993).

The foregoing discussion should serve as sufficient documentation that cross-cultural comparisons of the payments to family members for elder care is meaningless if the comparison does not take into account the total social welfare policy system of the countries being compared. The total sociocultural, political–ideological context determines whether payments to family caregivers will be considered a viable solution to caregiver shortages that beset countries with aging and old populations, or whether such payments are seen as a dangerous step toward undermining the altruistic nature of family relations. The United States falls clearly into the second category. Its particular constellation of institutional structures and cultural values provides a less than hospitable place for importing practices that have proven successful in Sweden, France, and Germany. The current consumer-direction movement with pilot projects for paying family caregivers or elders themselves to hire caregivers would take on a uniquely American character if it were to be implemented on a significant scale.

REFERENCES

Groger, L. (1984). State aid to peasants: Gifts or poison? A case-study from France. In O. M. Lynch (Ed.), *Culture and community in Europe: Essays in honor of Conrad M. Arensberg* (pp. 61–88). New Delhi: Hindustan Press.

Jani-Le Bris, H. (1993). *Family care of dependent older people in the European community*. Dublin, Ireland: European Foundation for the Improvement of Living and Working Conditions.

Linsk, N. L., Keigher, S. M., Simon-Rusinowitz, L. E., & England, S. E. (1992). *Wages for caring: Compensating family care of the elderly*. New York: Praeger.

Lechner, V. M., & Neal, M. B. (Eds.). (1999). *Work and caring for the elderly: International perspectives*. Philadelphia, PA: Brunner/Mazel.

Mauss, M. (1967). *The gift*. New York: Norton.

Montgomery, A., & Feinberg, L. F. (2003). *The road to recognition: International review of public policies to support family and informal caregiving*. San Francisco, CA: Family Caregiver Alliance.

Reichert, M., & Naegele, G. (1999). Elder care and the workplace in Germany: An issue for the future? In V. M. Lechner & M. B. Neal (Eds.), *Work and caring for the elderly: International perspectives* (pp. 29–46). Philadelphia, PA: Brunner/Mazel.

CHAPTER FIFTEEN

Response to Quality:

Differing Definitions

Elias S. Cohen

INTRODUCTION

Considering Quality of Care/Quality of Life

Four brief vignettes of life situations of elderly people with disabilities precede the body of this chapter. They are drawn from real life. I encountered these people and came to know them in different relationships—one over a lifetime, others in the course of research, and one over the course of several months. I visited the Lady on a Tether and the Lady Who Resigned in their homes in rural Pennsylvania in the course of a policy study on attendant care, and I explored, among other things, the relative importance and preference for consumer-directed care and agency-oriented programming. Alice the Collector was a client I represented (successfully) in a petition to have her competency restored. The Depressed Professor was a member of my extended family.

These life studies can serve to illustrate some of the complexity of the issues in identifying perspectives of the fact situation in any given situation, and the objective and subjective components of quality of care/quality of life circumstances. They are intended to assist the reader relate real lives to the abstract elements described in the chapter's main text.

RESPONSE TO QUALITY CASES

The Lady on a Tether

She was 86, and she suffered from pulmonary insufficiency secondary to coronary artery disease. She lived alone in her own home in a rural area in Central Pennsylvania. She was under the care of an internist, a cardiologist, and a pulmonary specialist from the hospital located about 20 miles from her home. She had no relatives living in the area or closer than 60 miles away. She received services from an Area Agency on Aging (AAA), which funded personal assistant (PA) care provided 3 hours a day every other day. The PA assisted with bathing and housekeeping, including laundry, food shopping, and some meal preparation. She was ambulatory, although dependent on nasal oxygen 24 hours a day. Large oxygen tanks were delivered to her home, and she had a 35-foot tube connected to the tank which allowed her to get anywhere in her house. She had not been outside her home in over a month. She was able to leave home only when she went to the hospital for a monthly medical visit and was accommodated by a paratransit service. She was adamant about wanting to stay in her own home, directing her attendant, and not going into a nursing home. She admitted to loneliness and missed being able to be outdoors, visiting, or going to church.

Alice the Collector

Alice, 85, lived alone on the outskirts of a small town near Gettysburg, Pennsylvania. I met her when I undertook having her competency restored. By any measure, Alice was eccentric. Her house was stuffed with things she had collected—newspapers, magazines, bottles, mason jars, and boxes of every size and description. She had somehow acquired what looked like warehouse shelving that took up all the wall space and area between. Her bedroom was piled high, and it was clear that she had left just enough room on the bed for her to curl around. The house had no toilet facilities, and neighbors complained that she dumped her slops in the garden, which, incidentally, seemed to flourish. The house was heated with a coal furnace; and the hot water, by a small coal furnace. Alice stoked the furnaces and removed the ashes. The house was in terrible repair—the gutters were falling down, the paint was peeling, and the porch looked dangerous.

Alice was in good physical health, having recovered from pneumonia, this illness gave rise to the appointment of a guardian to make health care decisions when she was unable to do so for herself. Alice's short-term memory was not great, and her narratives often confused time frames. She was slightly paranoid and was certain that important people had conspired to keep her from getting her Social Security checks—a charge which was not entirely true, but not entirely false either. Neither I nor the psychiatrist I retained (the former Pennsylvania Commissioner of Mental Health) believed that she was incompetent within the meaning of the law. We agreed that her judgment wasn't the best; nonetheless, she was clear about what she wanted, where she wanted it, and at least as important, what she didn't want.

We got her competency restored. We undertook to establish her eligibility for medical assistance and Supplemental Security Income to supplement her meager Social Security benefit. She indicated she wanted to fix up the house, and I arranged for her to receive a $5,000 to $10,000 grant plus a 30-year mortgage at 3%, which was manageable even with her small income.

Guess what! She turned it down. She didn't want to be in debt, and no cajoling or persuasion convinced her. In fact, she said I was stubborn. With those facts, I or anyone else could have gone back to the court to reinstate a guardian who would act in her best interest. But we didn't. We elected to respect her foolish decision, but we continued to offer her help, assistance, visits, transportation, and regular contact so long as she wanted it. Alice managed to stay in her home into her 90s when she became chronically ill and required substantial medical and nursing services, which could not be offered in her home.

The Depressed Professor

At 90, he lived alone in a lovely, well-furnished house that had been his home for 40 years. By any measure, he was economically well fixed with assets well in excess of $1 million and pension payments that exceeded his expenses. Widowed for the last 9 years, he maintained himself and the house in excellent condition. He had no children and lived about 250 miles from any family at all and about 400 miles from a brother from whom he had been estranged most of his life.

In the last year of living in his home, he lost most of his vision as a result of macular degeneration. His hearing was failing. In addition, he began to experience some difficulty in walking, although he was helped somewhat by use of a 4-foot cane. His mind was clear; his sense of humor, unchanged. At some point, apparently somewhat depressed, he took to staying in bed most of the day and night. His walking became increasingly problematic. Unknown to anyone, he had stopped taking thyroid and other medications. He had not seen his physician for about 5 months.

At some point, he called the woman who had been helping him with shopping for food and assisting in making out checks, to say that he was frightened of staying alone in his house. Through the assistance of a care manager, he was taken to an assisted living facility. There, he would get out of bed only to use his commode or the bathroom. He took his meals in his room on the edge of his bed. The care manager took him to his physician who did not recognize or acknowledge the depression that the Professor was experiencing. His problems were ascribed largely to old age. The Professor told some former colleagues who visited him that he was content to be in bed with his reveries. He refused to answer his phone or contact anyone—friends or family. He refused physical therapy designed to restore walking function. The case manager persuaded him to see a geriatric psychiatrist. Visits resulted in a diagnosis of depression and prescription of antidepressants. These improved his mood sufficiently, and he began some physical therapy and undertook walking and taking meals in the dining room, although he refused to have any contact with other residents. Those improvements notwithstanding, he continues to refuse to take or to make phone calls. He does not want anyone to assist with correspondence, and he has no interest in undertaking such himself. He refuses all assistive devices such as talking clocks, or assistance in learning to accommodate to his blindness. He disengages almost aggressively. His cognition is clear. Short-term memory is a problem, and occasionally he has problems in word finding. However, he has no problem discussing current events, although he refuses to listen to the radio or have readers for newspapers. Recently, he has taken to spending most of his time in bed, although his physical health is excellent and there are no disease processes going on.

The Lady Who Resigned

Widowed for 8 years, obese, arthritic, and seemingly either depressed or emotionally flat, she lived in her own home in a rural area. At 84, her principle problems involved her limited mobility and her lack of interest in anything except the mundane routines of everyday life. Her cognition did not appear impaired. She received limited attendant care at home to take care of housekeeping, laundry, bathing, and evening care. She had no desire to provide direction to her attendant, participate in scheduling, or suggest anything at all which she might find pleasing—not food, visits, going to church, or television. She did express that whatever her daughter arranged was fine with her. She did not express displeasure, confusion, or dissatisfaction with anything. Exercising choice was not her thing. What was, was.

QUALITY IS IN THE EYE OF THE BEHOLDER

Quality of long-term care, or perhaps more accurately *quality of life,* for the elderly or young, developmentally disabled and later-life disabled, cognitively impaired, and physically impaired alike, is like pornography—hard to describe precisely, but very recognizable. That said, we must quickly add that one man's Maplethorpe is another man's Larry Flynt.

Perhaps because such definitions are grounded in subjective interpretations, it is often difficult to come up with definitive measures and criteria. Controlling, influencing, and regulating pornography is very hard—and so is controlling, influencing, and regulating quality of long-term care and the quality of life for elderly persons with disabilities.

I want to approach the issue of definitions and reactions to them by looking at the issue of quality of care/quality of life broadly in the hope that in characterizing the "problems," the ensuing discussion will help broaden our approach to "solutions." There are five elements that I believe are relevant to a discussion on quality of care/quality of life:

1. Quality is in the eye of the beholder—Who are the beholders, and how broad or narrow is their vision?
2. What are the objective components of quality of care/quality of life, and are they sufficient to address the wishes/needs of the elderly disabled?
3. What are the subjective components of quality, and how do we think about them in the quest for quality?
4. What do we perceive as the critical barriers?
5. How do we proceed? We know how to solve the problem of quality for virtually any individual. The difficult question is: how do we do it 10,000 or 100,000 times while providing equal protection?

Key Beholders

Who are the key beholders? At a minimum, they include the older person with the disability; family and nonfamily caregivers; the state as guarantor of quality, often in the framework of its police power or in its *parens patriae* capacity to impose guardianships in the best interest of the incompetent (Horstman, 1975; Keith & Wacker, 1994); public and private third-party payers; and the community at large. Their respective views, although often conditioned by common factors, are not congruent. The beholders influence in various ways the quality-of-life outcomes for the elderly disabled individual. Some beholders are more determinative than others. The views and determinations of regulatory authorities may trump the conclusions and assessments of family. Third-party payers' views and determinations may trump the views of the person with a disability, and so on.

The critical view, particularly in the context of consumer direction, is the view of the elderly, who develop disability in their eighth and ninth decades of life and come to that new status with the baggage of previous generations—baggage which includes a crabbed view of old age referred to here as the elderly mystique. Let me take a few moments to review the phenomenon that I have described at greater length elsewhere (Cohen, 1988).

The elderly mystique, like the feminine mystique, refers to a view held by elderly persons themselves that potentials for growth, development, and continuing engagement virtually disappear when old age arrives. Rosalie Rosenfelt (1965), who first expressed the notion most eloquently over 40 years ago, concluded that the adherent of the mystique "knows society finds it hard to accept, let alone forgive his existence. An unsubtle attitude of punishment and retaliation is endemic in modern life. The old person expects derogation in explicit terms." Even earlier, Max Lerner (1957) wrote: "The culture (treats) the old like the fag end of what was once good material . . . the nicest thing you can say about an older American is that [he or she] 'doesn't look his age' and 'doesn't act his age'—as though it were the most damning thing in the world to look old."

Those comments were applied to the elderly in general and preceded the historically significant improvements in the physical and economic state of America's elderly people. The enormous progress in life expectancy, reduction of poverty, increased home ownership rates, higher net worth, and greater activity and participation in recreation and membership organizations all testify to the fact that old age "ain't what it used to be." And the negative elements of ageism, as viewed by the general population and the elderly themselves, have changed as well.

Instead of the earlier version of the mystique, which applied to all elderly people, I suggest that American ageism is now focused on the elderly with disabilities. Even the elderly themselves have concluded that when disability arrives, hope about continued growth, self-realization, and full participation in family and society must be abandoned so that all energy can be directed to avoiding the ultimate defeat, which is not death, but institutionalization, the equivalent of living death.

Furthermore, I suggest that waiver programs, demonstrations of consumer direction and consumer choice, and the minimal reduction in nursing home beds have not altered either the views of American society, in general, or the elderly population, in particular, in that regard. One has only to look at the explosion in assisted living facilities as evidence that we approve of, and the elderly find attractive the notions of colonies in which both external and internal supports are available for the price of giving up membership in the larger society.

None of this contradicts the persistence of the paradigm of biological inferiority—a marker of inferiority—applied to the elderly with disabilities. Our American tradition has held that compared to the dominant reference group, those who are regarded as biologically inferior are incapable of levels of self-fulfillment and self-realization and normal social participation, not to mention social contribution. Historically, five groups have been identified in these terms: people of color, the developmentally disabled, the physically disabled, the elderly disabled, and women.

Seen as impaired and vulnerable, the members of these groups require protection. As a result, those with beneficent inclinations and the members of the groups themselves set low goals, sometimes articulated and presented as high goals—for example, the least restrictive alternative. Historically, this set of beliefs has resulted in paternalistic perpetuation of roles and practices in which members have been held, or in which they have seen themselves, as diminished recipients of beneficence and paternalism, without high aspirations or even a sense that empowerment was a real possibility.

The last 40 years or so have seen enormous changes by and for African Americans, the developmentally disabled, the younger physically disabled identified with the Independent Living Movement, and women.

The elderly disabled, their families, caregivers and planners, and policymakers and practitioners, however, remain in the thrall of the elderly mystique.

Although the focus of prejudice against old age has shifted to prejudice against the elderly with disabilities, the roots are deep in our social psyche.

Popular music is the poetry of the common man (Cohen & Kruschwitz, 1990; Sohngen & Smith, 1978).[1] It is often a reflection of our sentimentalities, our idealizations, what we believe (or want to believe), what we prize, and what we fear. I hear America singing—singing about old age—for well over 100 years. The lyrics of these songs tell the

---

[1] For a treatment of aging in American popular sheet music, see Cohen and Kruschwitz (1990). Old age in America represented in nineteenth- and twentieth-century popular sheet music, *The Gerontologist, 30,* 345–354. See also Sohngen, M. and Smith, R. (1978). Images of old age in poetry, *The Gerontologist, 18,* 181–186.

tale, and often the titles alone speak volumes (for a treatment of aging in American popular sheet music, see Cohen & Kruschwitz,1990; see also Sohngen & Smith, 1978).

- Old age is a time of decline:

  "Old Joe Has Had His Day" (1912)

  The marks of time are creeping on
  My hair is turning grey
  The springtime of life has faded
  With the flow'rs that grow by the way
  We, like roses must wither and fade
  There's nothing comes to stay
  The allotted time is drawing near
  Old Joe has had his day

  "It's a Shame That We Have to Grow Old" (1917)

- Old age is a dismal time of life:

  "The Lone Old Man" (1858)
  "Only Waiting" (1864)
  "All the Grey Haired Men" (1968)
  "Old Friends" (1968)

  "Why Chime the Bells So Merrily?" (1835)

- To be old is to be abandoned:

  "Over the Hill to the Poorhouse" (1874)

  For I'm old and I'm helpless and feeble,
  The days of my youth have gone by.
  Then over the hill to the poorhouse,
  I wander alone there to die.

- Old Age is a time of loss of attractiveness:

  "Get Away, Old Man, Get Away" (1927)

  Don't ever marry an old man
  I'll tell you the reason why
  His lips are all tobacco juice
  His chin is never dry

For an old man he is grey,
But a young man's heart is full of love,
Get away, old man, get away

"Will You Love Me When I'm Old?" (1873)

"Will You Love Me When My Face Is Worn and Old?" (1907)

- The Good Life is for the young; it was better when I was vigorous, lusty, and energetic:

  "O Would I Were a Boy Again" (1850)

  "Past Days Are Dear" (1865)

  "If I Could Call the Years Back" (1907)

  "When You and I Were Young, Maggie" (1910)

- The goal—Eternal youth:

  "I Wish I Was Eighteen Again" (1978), George Burns's signature piece.

  "At the Fountain of Youth" (1915)

This brief excursion is hardly an in-depth inquiry into the perceptions of late-life disability, beliefs, and roles. To be sure, there is evidence of these perceptions reflected in the raw material of numbers of skilled nursing facility beds, assisted living facility beds, personal care attendant service utilization by the elderly, marketing surveys, and other quantitative measures, although those are not apt to provide significant clues about *beliefs* and *images* of what people with disabilities regard as successful old age. However, they offer clues about the operative values that underpin the views of beholders of disability in old age. To the extent that they reflect generally held views, they affect the views of the elderly themselves and the views of their family and nonfamily caregivers.

There is a serious disconnect between the articulated views of consumers and their caregivers and what is effectively communicated to the marketplace, the legislature, and the executive branch agencies. In Pennsylvania, for example, an inquiry in 1997 sought the opinions of consumers, providers of long-term care, and advocates for people with disabilities about the long-term care system and the values that were salient. The inquiry was conducted through a dozen focus groups conducted throughout the commonwealth. Three values common to *all* participants were identified: "(1) Remain independent and live at home as long as possible,

(2) respect and dignity for the individual, [and] (3) consumer choice." A major conclusion was the "belief that the funding system, the philosophies which guide it, and the regulations which drive it are outdated and out of touch with consumers' needs . . . [and that] the system is so broken that it cannot be fixed. [The informants] want the system to be rethought, redesigned and redirected" (Pennsylvania Intra-Governmental Council on Long-Term Care, 1997).

Yet, in spite of the passion, and the apparent unanimity, not only is there little articulation about what quality of long-term care looks like and what quality old age with disability looks like, but also there is little effective demand for care which embodies the three common values: life in one's own home, respect and dignity, and consumer direction. The report states that Pennsylvania allocated 77% of its long-term care and services dollars for nursing facilities and 23% for home- and community-based care. And further, that there were 8,000 Pennsylvanians waiting for a variety of community-based services—and my guess is that a very small proportion of those were elderly.

Why is that? My hunch is that there is a widely held view, which translates into widespread reliance on nursing homes and lack of belief in community-based services, that when disability comes to the elderly, there is no real future, participation is a lost cause, the trajectory is inexorably downhill, and we should not expect very much in the way of successful outcomes. The result is a grudging acquiescence to institutionalization.

THE OBJECTIVE COMPONENTS OF QUALITY LONG-TERM CARE

What is left then? For the state, the ultimate protector, it is the assurance of safety, cleanliness, attention to physical arrangements and medical needs, pleasant surroundings, freedom from too much inhumane care, and assurance of quality components that can be objectively measured. And this is the view that many caregivers bring to the business of long-term care. And judging from the nature of journalistic exposés and well-meaning articles about long-term care, it is what families and the community at large are concerned with. However, even that concern is limited and does not fully protect long-term care recipients from other forms of bodily or psychic insult. We can count the number of people in nursing homes or who receive community-based services with depression—if it is recognized, and it often is not. So where is the quality of care in a facility where 25% of the residents present with depression (Joiner, Pettit, & Perez, 2002), in my opinion, most of it untreated? What is the quality standard for care of people with dementing illness? Do we even seek to increase the moments of joy, of pleasure, of satisfaction, much less measure it? Or are we inclined to believe that dementia is the ultimate insult, robbing the person of even the capability of being pleased, and therefore, because memory is gone, we need not even try to enhance the quality of life?

What beholders see, what they believe, what their interests and biases are, all influence what they measure and what they overlook. Consequently, the measures define what services, accommodations, utilities, and relationships we provide and support.

We have constricted our vision about quality of life and quality of care for the elderly with disabilities. Measuring safety, creature comforts, nutrition, and all the things we regulate is relatively easy. However, providers can meet every official requirement and still fall short of quality care that enhances the quality of life. We can measure the nature and impact of disease and disability on the individual, and, unless we believe that interventions are futile, we specify and measure the nature of commensurate ameliorative actions. Objective measures are important and useful in setting some bare legal minimums. They are necessary but insufficient. It is the moral imperative that governs "please" and "thank you," and respectful speech and body language, and the constant quest to maximize and validate individual qualities even when disability may limit some kinds of social participation.

Would it have been possible to be more creative in addressing the issues confronting us in the matter of the Depressed Professor? (See "life studies, p. 234–236.) Or was it already too late? And what might we have done, if we had the opportunity 6 or 12 months earlier? How creative and expansive are we in the search for enhancing the quality of life for the elderly with disabilities?

To what extent do we routinely provide systematic housing assessments to determine what accommodations might render housing more hospitable to the disabled elder? To what extent do we extend services to assist elderly individuals to accommodate to their blindness, or deafness, or other sensory deficits? To what extent do we retrofit automobiles with hand controls for those with hip or leg problems? Do we evaluate and intervene where depression, disengagement, and despair have produced massive disability? Or do we even know how to establish a baseline for an individual so that we can determine normative levels of socialization, engagement with a larger community, or even such simple things as whether being outdoors is pleasurable or not. And these are the easy elements. In other words, what do we know about figuring out what is important in the life of the older person with a disability?

SUBJECTIVE COMPONENTS OF QUALITY
LONG-TERM CARE

It gets harder the more we begin to explore the subjective components of quality. I take as my initiating texts Bart Collopy's (1988) seminal article and an earlier unpublished report of his (1986).

Collopy (1988) suggests that the "relentless logic of elderly diminishment" is yoked to the perception of long-term care for the elderly. Notions of autonomy "counter the paternalistic tendencies of medicine and social services as well as the cultural stereotypes which assign the elderly to passivity and homogeneity" and challenge the "automatic and untested use of 'best interests' or patient welfare arguments to override elderly self-determination."

"Self-determination," "Consumer choice," "Consumer voice," "Consumer-direction," and "consumer orientation" are all terms, which take their meaning from our understanding of the notion of autonomy. Collopy (1988, p. 11) lays out for us six polarities, which are embodied in the notion. Each of these deserves attention when dealing with real lives. The case studies referred to below are presented at the beginning of this chapter.

- Decisional Versus Executional: Having preferences, making decisions versus being able to implement them or carry them out. Each of the case studies involves the distinction.
- Direct Versus Delegated: Deciding or acting on one's own versus giving authority to others to decide/act. The Lady who resigned delegated everything. Should we be comfortable with that? Or are we bound by her decisions?
- Competent Versus Incapacitated: Reasonably and judgmentally coherent choice/activity versus that which exhibits rational defect or judgmental incoherence. What about Alice the Collector? How would we know if she "stepped over the line"?
- Authentic Versus Inauthentic: Choices/actions that are consonant with character versus those which are seriously out of character. Each case raises the question. Was the Lady Who Resigned always authentically acquiescing, or was her view jaded by her disability?
- Immediate Versus Long Range: Present or limited expressions of autonomy versus future or wide-ranging expressions. Alice took the long view—perhaps unrealistically although always infused with optimism. The Depressed Professor, did just the opposite.

- Negative Versus Positive: Choice/activity that claims a right only to noninterference versus that which claims positive entitlement, support, capacitation. Which does each of the studies represent?

Collopy also points out that although these polarities are useful in understanding elder autonomy, lives are more complex than these categories suggest. Crucial aspects of autonomy—independence and individuality—don't take into account sufficiently realistic notions of participation and reciprocity among family, friends, caregivers, agencies, organizations, and others. How people participate with each other; how they reciprocate; what is autonomous, and what is distinguished from resignation, acquiescence, acceptance, affirmative compliance, delegation and authenticity are subtle and always subject to interpretation.

These subtleties are important because narrow applications of self-determination and consumer direction may mask the exercise of autonomy and obliterate some important elements of life satisfaction in important domains. To the extent that "staying in one's own home" trumps everything else, there may be a result that increases isolation, reduces participation in community, neighborhood, and family, and perhaps worst of all, conveyance to consumers that "the least restrictive alternative" is the highest goal, when in fact, it may be a perversion of the desideratum—"the most liberating alternative."

In its most expansive sense, self-determination and all of its derivatives always support a sense of self, a life view by the individual. This, in turn, requires the conviction that people with disabilities, with severe disabilities whether physical or cognitive, *have* a life view—that they have the capacity to flourish, to engage, to experience joy, satisfaction, contentment, and their opposites. And this requires the recognition that each moment is precious, each moment is an opportunity to flourish, to engage, to experience joy—whether or not it is remembered in the next moment, or whether it is experienced in ways different from the ways that you or I understand the moment.

CRITICAL BARRIERS

Elsewhere, James Conroy (e.g., Center for Outcome Analysis, 2001) has described the success we have enjoyed not only in the fact of increasing self-determination in developmental disability (DD) programming but also in our ability to evaluate outcomes. Surely the same definitional issues of measurement of objective and subjective components confronted programmers and evaluators in DD that we now confront in aging.

Well, maybe. I believe the barriers are different.

I have dwelt on one already—at length. The elderly mystique and its constricted view of the quality of life and the prospects for high quality when disability is a reality of old age stands in the way of securing the benefits of self-determination and the exercise of consumer choice. Examples of the mystique are rife. They are found not so much in affirmative statements about how futile quality is when disability strikes as in the images of "successful agers" and in the absence of descriptions of high-quality aging in the presence of disability.

The recent publication by Rowe and Kahn (1998) presents the findings of the MacArthur Foundation study on how lifestyle choices determine your health and vitality. It is silent about "successful aging" with a disability. It is entirely about preserving health, preserving roles, and preserving activity so that one comes to old age in better shape. But if one doesn't, does that constitute "failure"? According to Holstein and Minkler (2003) there is a danger that we exaggerate the extent to which these decisions, and the knowledge and resources they require, are equally available to all older people. It is the notion that failure is the inescapable consequence of old age, and particularly the failure of disability in old age that is at the heart of the elderly mystique. The power of the mystique is pervasive because it is most strongly held by the elderly and those who care for and about them.

Worthy of address as a barrier are the constrained views of those who are most influential and who participate in the social policy process: program administrators, legislators, legislative staffers, practitioners including lawyers, doctors, social workers, financial planners, fiduciaries, regulators, and ethicists. Too many of us are defining the elephant with limited perspectives.

We are enamored of slogans and silver bullets:

- If only Medicaid shifted its emphasis.
- If only consumer direction and self determination were the absolute rule.
- If only the dictates of *Olmstead*[2] (1999) were honored.
- If only we closed the nursing homes and the intermediate care facilities.
- If only regulation lived up to its vaunted goals.

---

[2] *Olmstead v. L.C.*, 527 U.S. (1999), the U.S. Supreme Court Case which held that states may be violating title II of the Americans with Disabilities Act if they provide care to people with disabilities in institutional settings when they could be appropriately served in a home or community based setting.

- If only the elderly took better care of themselves.
- If only the elderly and their families were politically energized and organized.
- If only the scourge of ageism were eradicated.
- If only poverty in old age were eliminated.

This is the silver-bullet trap. It is difficult to avoid in refashioning human services. We—I have been a participant along with other advocates and social planners in the failure to address systematically the mechanisms of massive social change and to affect effectively the power configurations that control problem solving. The history of our mistakes in using the silver bullet approach is a long one:

The "fix up" strategy initially promoted in mental health and mental retardation.

The separation of financial assistance and social services in public assistance programs under the Social Security Act.

The wholesale reliance on case management for social service delivery and control.

Managed care for health service delivery.

Protective legislation for women intended to free them from the hazards of traditional male occupations because of their inherent biological inferiority.

Separate but equal facilities and services for people of color.

The silver-bullet approach, the failure to understand the meaning of autonomy, the elderly mystique—these are the real barriers—more real than inadequate appropriations, more real than the insufficient manpower considerations, more real than the absence of cures and amelioratives, and more real than economic determinism.

The barriers all stem from the differing perceptions, differing definitions of quality of life, quality of service, and our misreading the nature of outcomes from various interventions. And that should tell us what we have to do.

Our task, I believe, is nothing less than to construct quality-of-life definitions for all—not only for the young, the middle aged, the educated, the healthy, and the well-to-do but also for the old, the sick, the dropout, and the disabled.

Doing this requires the design of various strategies including legislative and legal, research and education, market, service delivery, and community organizing. It will not be accomplished by reforming current agency-dominated health care assessment and delivery services alone, although that is a critical component. Doubling or quadrupling these will not accomplish it, nor will massive extension of waiver programs—doing that will more likely reinforce the notion that inpatient care is the default service, when what we need is precisely the opposite. We should require states to secure waivers for long-term inpatient care (in effect limiting institutional care), and for community-based services to have the open-ended funding.

It will not be accomplished by increasing Social Security or Supplemental Security Income payment levels, although eliminating poverty as we currently define it would help.

Silver-bullet approaches are siren seductresses that show lots of promise, but are disastrous in the delivery. Neither utopia nor paradise follows the silver bullet.

Like Edgar Allen Poe's short story, "The Purloined Letter," the answer is here before us in plain sight. It is through convocations that bring together those working with the problems and issues and people every day, who struggle using the tools they have to find solutions. It will take lawyers, sociologists, administrators, social workers, and health care professionals who are willing to stretch their minds, abandon what is comfortable and knowable, and join to resolve the complex problems with elegant solutions. With imagination, resolve, and courage, we can fashion and deliver solutions to virtually any individual problematic life situation and offer the highest quality of life consistent with the capacities of the disabled person.

The hard part is how to do this 10,000 or a 100,000 times.

REFERENCES

Center for Outcome Analysis. (2001). *Personal life quality protocol—California quality tracking project, version 10.2*, Narbeth, PA.

Cohen, E. S. (1988). The elderly mystique: Constraints on the autonomy of the elderly with disabilities. *The Gerontologist, 28*(Suppl.), 24–31.

Cohen, E. S., & Kruschwitz, A. L. (1990). Old age in America represented in nineteenth and twentieth century popular sheet music. *The Gerontologist, 30*, 345–354.

Collopy, B. J. (1986). *The conceptually problematic status of autonomy*. Study prepared for the Retirement Research Foundation (unpublished).

Collopy, B. J. (1988). Autonomy in long-term care: some crucial distinctions. *The Gerontologist, 28*(Suppl.), 10–17.

Horstman, P. M. (1975). Protective services for the elderly: The limits of parens patriae. *Missouri, 40*, 215–278.

Holstein, M. B., & Minkler, M. (2003). Self, society and the "new gerontology." *The Gerontologist, 43*, 787–796.

Joiner, T. E., Pettit, J. W., & Perez, M. (2002). Depression. In D. Eckerdt (Ed.), *Encyclopedia of aging* (p. 336). New York: MacMillan.

Keith, P. M., & Wacker, R. R. (1994). *Older wards and their guardians.* Westport, CT: Praeger.

Lerner, M. (1957). *America as a civilization.* New York: Simon & Schuster.

Olmstead v. L.C., 527 U.S. (1999).

Pennsylvania Intra-Governmental Council on Long-Term Care. (1997). *Long-term care and services: Discussion session findings*, Harrisburg, PA.

Rosenfelt, R. (1965). The elderly mystique. *Journal of Social Issues, 21*, 37–43.

Rowe, J. W., & Kahn, R. L. (1998). *Successful Aging*, New York: Pantheon Press.

Sohngen, M., & Smith, R. (1978). Images of old age in poetry. *The Gerontologist, 18*, 181–186.

CHAPTER SIXTEEN

When Consumer Direction Fails:

Assigning Legal and Ethical Responsibility in Worst-Case Situations

Marshall B. Kapp

In most cases, the emerging consumer-direction paradigm (Stone, 2000) is likely to improve the quality of care and quality of life for chronically disabled individuals who need various types of long-term care (LTC). In some situations, however, this paradigm will fail and an awful set of circumstances may materialize (e.g., headlines announcing 90-year-old woman found confused, filthy, and emaciated in her apartment because she used her government-provided home care voucher to buy food for her 18 cats rather than food, medicine, and services for herself). Such worst-case scenarios implicate a panoply of legal and ethical concerns for all the involved parties. Agencies coordinating home- and community-based (HCB) LTC programs that incorporate elements of consumer direction are particularly concerned about their exposure to potential legal liability and ethical criticism if worst-case scenarios erupt. This chapter aims to identify and briefly discuss key issues associated with these legal and ethical anxieties. Dealing proactively with these apprehensions about an unacceptable dichotomy between accountability and control is a task that is essential, if we are to translate our lofty philosophical commitment to consumer direction into a practical, functioning system that implements the values undergirding this relatively new approach to LTC.

ELEMENTS OF A NEGLIGENCE CLAIM

A logical way to commence a discussion of agency fears about liability risks associated with consumer-directed LTC is by outlining the four essential elements that a plaintiff must prove in a professional malpractice lawsuit based, as the vast majority of such claims are, on a theory of negligence (i.e., unintentional but blameworthy wrongdoing; Showalter, 1999, pp. 43–57). To a significant extent, parallels may be drawn between these legal elements and relevant ethical questions.

The *first element* that a plaintiff must prove in a negligence action is that there was a duty of due care owed by the defendant to the plaintiff. Normally, this duty arises out of a special relationship existing between the parties. In the consumer-direction context, whether an agency owes a duty of due care to the consumer depends on the existence and nature of the contractual or fiduciary (Kapp, 1995, pp. 31–32) relationship formed between the agency and the consumer. Precisely what duty is owed is defined by the applicable standard of care, which is "reasonable" conduct in the circumstances as determined by the ordinary conduct of the defendant's prudent, competent peers. There have been no reported legal opinions dealing particularly with the standard of care that agencies owe consumers under consumer-directed LTC models, so early cases in this arena will need to draw on common law precedent that has developed in analogous areas through a process of case-by-case adjudication. It is important to keep in mind that the duty of care to be expected of an agency, even when the agency stands in a fiduciary relationship with the consumer, is—under present tort law principles—limited to protecting against risks that could be reasonably foreseen and averted or mitigated.

The *second element* of proof in a negligence action is a breach or violation by the defendant of the duty owed to the plaintiff. This is the requirement, under present tort law, of fault. Attention to this element ought to encourage agencies to prospectively formulate plans for satisfying their duties, while taking into account available, reasonable alternatives or options that are least restrictive of, and least intrusive into, consumers' right to control the details of their own care. An open question at this time is the extent to which an agency may legally and ethically shift part of its duty to a consumer who voluntarily and knowingly agrees to accept and assume the possible consequences of the consumer's risky choices;

respect for consumer autonomy argues for a broad application of the assumption of risk doctrine here. On the other hand, some might not only oppose allowing agencies to limit their accountability through the assumption of risk doctrine but also contend further that the fault element be eliminated in this context and strict or absolute liability be imposed in its stead; such a public policy approach would effectively make agencies administering consumer-directed programs the insurers of good results for the consumer.

Third, a plaintiff seeking to establish a negligence claim must present evidence of damage or injury. The damage or injury in a negligence claim usually involves tangible, demonstrable physical and/or emotional harm. However, one way to characterize damage in the consumer-direction context may be as a failure to achieve a goal that should have been achieved as part of the administering agency's duty of care. This begs the issue of identifying which goal or goals have been agreed on by the parties as paramount within a particular agency/consumer relationship, because the potential goals of safety (embodying the ethical precept of nonmaleficence), freedom of choice (predicated on the ethical principle of autonomy), and maximization of consumer potential (based on the idea of beneficence, or doing good) may conflict in particular situations (Kane & Levin, 1998).

A link of proximate, or the most direct, causation between the defendant's violation of duty and the plaintiff's injury is the *fourth element* that must be established in negligence litigation. An agency could be held responsible for injury suffered by a consumer only to the extent that the consumer's own choices and actions failed to break the causal link between agency negligence and consumer injury. This factor again raises questions about the proper applicability of the assumption of risk and contributory negligence doctrines as defenses against agency liability in this context (Furrow, Greaney, Johnson, Jost, & Schwartz, 2000, pp. 294–297). The legal outcome in specific situations probably would depend on whether the consumer's own risky behaviors, or different external forces that were influencing the outcomes of LTC for the consumer, were or were not reasonably foreseeable and controllable by the administrative agency.

In light of the foregoing analytic framework, we can next consider in more particularity some legal and ethical issues regarding the duties arguably owed to consumers by agencies that are coordinating publicly funded, consumer-directed LTC programs, namely: is there a duty (and the authority) to limit who can be a "consumer," and, if so, what does such a duty entail? Is there a duty (and a right) to limit various aspects of the "choice" that is available to participants in consumer-directed LTC programs?

IS THERE A DUTY (AND AUTHORITY) TO LIMIT
WHO CAN BE A "CONSUMER"?

Both current and proposed eligibility criteria for the receipt of publicly
financed HCB LTC services are based on two factors: (1) the individual's
level of physical and/or mental impairment or need for health and human services and (2) the individual's financial need for public support
(i.e., a financial means-test). Introducing the concept of consumer direction compels us to investigate a third eligibility criterion, specifically, the
consumer's capacity to choose and direct his or her own LTC plan (Kapp,
1999). If consumer capacity is deemed essential to the autonomous exercise of consumer direction, there must be some responsibility to assess
each consumer candidate in this regard. Such an obligation suggests several questions.

First, how should a minimally adequate level of decisional capacity
be defined in this context in functional, decision-specific terms? What
precise kinds and degrees of cognitive and emotional abilities must a
person demonstrate to be considered capable enough to make independent choices about the details (the who, when, where, and how) of
his or her own LTC plan, especially if (as will almost always be true)
some of those choices entail foreseeable and preventable risks to the
consumer?

Second, how should the process of capacity assessment work logistically? Who has the duty to conduct an assessment—the agency administering the consumer-directed LTC program, individual service providers,
both, or someone else? When is there a responsibility to initiate the involvement of experts to conduct formal assessments instead of relying on
the working judgment of case managers and clinicians in the field made
"on the fly"? At what point(s) in the enrollment and service delivery process should formal or informal capacity assessments occur? When is it
necessary to use formal capacity assessment instruments, and how much
weight should be placed on the results produced by those instruments
in supplementing or supplanting the practical intuition and experience
of case managers and clinicians (Kapp & Mossman, 1996)? Do there
even exist written instruments that are specifically designed to assess a
person's capacity for consumer direction of LTC and, if not, should instruments for this purpose be developed? When, if ever, and why should
the issue of a candidate consumer's decisional capacity be referred to a
court of law for official adjudication, and who ought to initiate judicial
involvement?

Finally, how ought administrative agencies and service providers account for the fact that, although a consumer theoretically always retains
the right to change his or her mind about the details of the LTC plan or to

withdraw from the plan completely, in reality the consumer's decisional capacity may deteriorate over time to an extent that would make subsequent decisions nonautonomous? Put differently, how do we protect a consumer's ongoing right to choose while acknowledging the possibility of that same consumer's cognitive and emotional downward slide? Is there a duty to assess capacity continuously and, if so, how should that duty be fulfilled reasonably and practically?

When consumers lack sufficient capacity to autonomously direct their own LTC, proxy decision makers become involved. In many situations, even when adequate decisional capacity on the consumer's part is present, the consumer may wish to have decisions about the details of the LTC plan made in a shared or joint arrangement with his or her family, rather than in an isolated, atomistic fashion by himself or herself (Kapp, 1991). The phenomena of proxy and/or joint decision making implicates a variety of issues for the administrative agency and individual LTC providers in a (misnamed) consumer-directed model (Cicirelli, 1992; Kapp, 2001).

For instance, in what circumstances should (or must) an administering agency or provider insist that there be formal legal authority held by the proxy or joint decision maker (e.g., created by execution of a durable power of attorney document or a judicial guardianship order) instead of accepting the informal sharing or delegation of authority arrangements much more commonly found in the HCB LTC context? When the authority of a proxy is made contingent on the consumer's loss of sufficient decisional capacity (as it usually is in a durable power of attorney), who has the obligation to determine when that contingency has occurred, and by what process? To what standards of decision making should proxies be held by the agencies and providers who will carry out their decisions of substituted judgment (i.e., standing in the consumer's shoes to the extent that the consumer's authentic contemporary wishes can be ascertained or inferred), the proxy's judgment about the consumer's best interests, some combination of the two, or a different test?

In situations involving proxy or shared decision making, the administering agency and particular providers may confront legal and ethical challenges in sorting out and reconciling conflicting loyalties and responsibilities owed to the disabled consumer, on one hand, and the consumer's family members, on the other. Family members, after all, have morally legitimate interests of their own that may be placed at serious jeopardy by the demands imposed on their finite time, energies, and finances by the consumer's service needs. From a strictly pragmatic perspective, few HCB LTC plans can work effectively without substantial family cooperation. Thus, answering the question—"Who is the consumer or client?; that is, to whom are legal and ethical duties owed (Monson, 1993)—often is not as straightforward a proposition as might appear at first blush.

IS THERE A DUTY (AND AUTHORITY) TO LIMIT "CHOICE" WITHIN THE CONSUMER CHOICE MODEL?

To be meaningful beyond its rhetorical value, the concept of consumer choice assumes that the consumer will have available an array of different alternatives from which to select. However, a number of forces, for example, legal and ethical as well as financial, and the realities of the labor pool (Noelker, 2001) combine to limit the range of choices actually available to any particular consumer.

To satisfy its legal and ethical responsibilities, must (or at least may) an agency administering a consumer-directed LTC program place reasonable restrictions on *who* a consumer may employ to deliver services? More specifically, is the agency, as a matter of protecting the consumer against potential harm (i.e., nonmaleficence), required or at least permitted to partially constrict consumer autonomy by imposing structural requirements (such as professional licensure, certification, or registration or periodic testing for drug use) or structural disqualifications (such as the presence of a criminal record) as preconditions for being hired by the consumer? Whom, if anyone, is it proper to expose to legal liability or moral censure if such preconditions are not set and a provider accidentally or intentionally injures a consumer?

In response to the "Who may be hired?" question, consumers in many consumer-directed HCB LTC programs are permitted to hire independent providers (IPs). Who has the responsibility to assure the rights of an IP regarding such matters as compliance with minimum wage and hour laws; health, life, and disability insurance; pension; vacation and sick time; workers' compensation coverage; and payment of FICA and other taxes?

Furthermore, does the administering agency have the power, or at least permission, to intrude on unbridled consumer autonomy by placing boundaries on *the specific kinds of services* that consumers might choose to purchase under the publicly funded HCB LTC program? As a matter of public policy, isn't there some duty to taxpayers to make the purchase with public dollars of certain services (e.g., cable television with premium channels) out of bounds even if the consumer wants them? Moreover, cannot the setting of limits be justified or even mandated in the name of beneficence and nonmaleficence when consumer choices (e.g., to spend one's public allotment on cat food rather than on food or medication for oneself) threaten to become manifestations of self-neglect? How imminent and serious must the threat of harm be to justify benevolent intrusion?

Operating within whatever limits may be established in a consumer-directed LTC program regarding what services may be chosen and by whom they may be provided, what is the extent of the administering agency's duty to assure that the choices made by consumers and/or their proxies and collaborators are *informed and voluntary*? Having the necessary information and exercising free volition in decision making (along with mental capacity, discussed already) are the key elements necessary if decisions are to be characterized as legally and morally valid (Faden & Beauchamp, 1986). Who has the responsibility to disclose to the consumer or proxy sufficient material information about available choices and to assure that the consumer or proxy effectively comprehends the disclosed information? Pragmatically speaking, how should information be presented, and by what standard (i.e., from the perspective of the ordinary program administrator or service provider versus that of the reasonable consumer) should the adequacy of the information be judged? In the realm of voluntariness, what is the obligation, and who owes it, under the principle of social or distributive justice to advocate on the macro level for and facilitate the availability of sufficient acceptable choices for the consumer? Is a forced selection from among unattractive options truly an exercise of "voluntary" choice?

In consumer-directed LTC models, effective quality assurance efforts may impinge on consumer choices that might otherwise entail the consumer tolerating the risk or reality of poor quality services. The specific goals of quality oversight mechanisms (e.g., safety vs. maximizing autonomy) would directly affect where lines get drawn, in terms of degree of risk tolerated. The proper division of responsibility for quality assurance between the program coordinating agency and particular service providers needs to be clearly worked out in advance. When interventions motivated by quality assurance objectives are undertaken in the face of consumer protests, they must be guided by the least intrusive or least restrictive alternative principle, that is, intruding on the individual consumer's right to choose only to the extent necessary to accomplish the legitimate goals of the intervention (Kapp, 1995, p. 43). Also, those who design and effectuate quality assurance efforts must take into account the privacy interests of consumers and develop management systems that protect as assiduously as feasible the confidentiality of information that could identify particular persons.

TENSION BETWEEN RISK MANAGEMENT AND ETHICS

Quite understandably, agencies coordinating consumer-directed programs as well as the agencies and individuals who provide direct services within consumer-directed models often incur serious anxieties regarding potentially negative legal, ethical, financial, and public consequences associated with worst-case scenarios of severe consumer abuse or neglect. It certainly is ethically appropriate for agencies and providers to be concerned with their own, as well as their client's, realistic risks; an agency or provider that is severely hobbled financially or otherwise because of adverse legal or media repercussions cannot effectively serve anyone. Unfortunately, these apprehensions frequently create a perceived (sometimes accurate but often exaggerated or misplaced) tension between good risk management practices and respect for the ethical principle of consumer autonomy (Kapp, 1998). As much as possible, coordinating agencies and service providers ought to recognize the ethical costs of excessive or misdirected risk management strategies and work toward maximizing the synergistic effects of risk management and a commitment to consumer autonomy (as well as beneficence).

Agencies and providers might pursue a number of proactive strategies, both individually and collectively, toward accomplishing such a synergy. The practical workability of *negotiated risk contracts* agreed to by all involved parties is one avenue to be explored (Kapp & Wilson, 1995). Working together, agencies that administer consumer-directed LTC programs could develop and disseminate consensus *industry practice guidelines or protocols* addressing many of the foreseeable problems likely to be encountered in consumer-directed LTC models; compliance with such guidelines or protocols may be beneficial both in improving the quality of professional practice and as evidence in a lawsuit that the agency or provider acted within the acceptable standard of care (Rosoff, 2001). Leaders in the consumer-direction movement, representing the academic, health care, and social services communities, should actively identify and publicize contemporary Best Practices. These Best Practices should positively reconcile agency and provider risk management interests with promotion of consumer prerogatives, so that others may emulate those exemplars. Each agency and provider should create and adopt written policies and procedures that are consistent with industry guidelines but attuned and adapted to the particular circumstances, resources, and consumer-directed model(s) pertinent to that specific agency or provider.

A related, ongoing, and essential strategy is to educate agency staff, service providers, consumers, families, regulators, and consumer advocates about the legal and ethical issues and principles discussed in this chapter, including any relevant industry guidelines and particular agency or provider policies and procedures. At the least, a shared vocabulary, sensitized participants, open lines of communication, and a common conceptualization of key challenges and values can go far to foster positive relationships that help avoid or mitigate potential conflicts that might otherwise escalate into recriminations and litigation in those relatively rare but real situations in which the consumer choice model of LTC fails and worst-case scenarios occur.

Finally, when confronted with legal and ethical ambiguities and apprehensions, there still seems to be a widely accepted tendency to assume that enactment of even more legislation and/or regulation is somehow the best route to removing those ambiguities and calming those apprehensions. Experience in a variety of contexts largely disproves this assumption (Howard, 2001). Amendments to current statutes and regulations should be advocated only very selectively and judiciously, when less drastic alternatives have been considered but rejected. The kinds of voluntary initiatives outlined previously are much more likely to achieve the desired objectives of melding good legal risk management with the ethical values that undergird the long overdue paradigm shift toward greater consumer choice and direction in LTC.

REFERENCES

Cicirelli, V. G. (1992). *Family caregiving: Autonomous and paternalistic decision making*. Newbury Park, CA: Sage.

Faden, R. R., & Beauchamp, T. L. (1986). *A history and theory of informed consent*. New York: Oxford University Press.

Furrow, B. R., Greaney, T. L., Johnson, S. H., Jost, T. S., & Schwartz, R. L. (2000). *Health law* (2nd ed.). St. Paul, MN: West Group.

Howard, P. K. (2001). *The lost art of drawing the line: How fairness went too far*. New York: Random House.

Kane, R. A., & Levin, C. A. (Fall 1998). Who's safe? Who's sorry? The duty to protect the safety of clients in home- and community-based care. *Generations, 22*(3), 76–81.

Kapp, M. B. (2001). Consumer choice in home- and community-based long-term care: Policy implications for decisionally incapacitated consumers. *Home Health Care Services Quarterly, 19*(4), 17–50.

Kapp, M. B. (1999). Health care in the marketplace: Implications for decisionally impaired consumers and their surrogates and advocates. *Southern Illinois University Law Journal, 24*, 1–51.

Kapp, M. B. (1991). Health care decision making by the elderly: I get by with a little help from my family. *Gerontologist, 31*, 619–623.

Kapp, M. B. (1995). *Key words in ethics, law, and aging: A guide to contemporary usage*. New York: Springer Publishing Company.

Kapp, M. B. (1998). *Our hands are tied: Legal tensions and medical ethics*. Westport, CT: Auburn House.

Kapp, M. B., & Mossman, D. (1996). Measuring decisional capacity: Cautions on the construction of a "capacimeter." *Psychology, Public Policy, and Law, 2*, 73–95.

Kapp, M. B., & Wilson, K. B. (1995). Assisted living and negotiated risk: Reconciling protection and autonomy. *Journal of Ethics, Law, and Aging, 1,* 5–13.

Monson, T. (1993). Perspective from Minnesota. In R. A. Kane & A. L. Caplan (Eds.), *Ethical conflicts in the management of home care: The case manager's dilemma* (pp. 76–78). New York: Springer.

Noelker, L. S. (Guest Ed.). (2001). Who will care for older people? Workforce issues in a changing society [Theme issue]. *Generations, 25*(1), 1–94.

Rosoff, A. J. (2001). Evidence-based medicine and the law: The courts confront clinical practice guidelines. *Journal of Health Politics, Policy, & Law, 26,* 327–368.

Showalter, J. S. (1999). *The law of healthcare administration* (3rd ed.). Chicago: Health Administration Press.

Stone, R. I. (Guest Ed.). (2000). Consumer direction in long-term care [Theme issue]. *Generations, 24*(3).

Index

Page numbers followed by f indicate figure; those followed by t indicate table.

261